"*The Pain Management Workbook* is an unmatched resource ... ook is written in an easily comprehensible, conversational style that is unlike any other, and fills a huge void in the understanding of pain. Rachel Zoffness's book will become a standard text offering millions of pain sufferers the tools to manage their pain."

—**Jack Stern, MD, PhD**, professor of neurosurgery at New York Medical College; author of *Ending Back Pain*; editorial review board member of *Spine* and *The Spine Journal*; and past president of the board of governors at Albert Einstein College of Medicine

"This book challenges the reader to take a science-based, potentially transformative journey toward recovery from chronic pain, surely one of the most burdensome health problems we face. Rachel Zoffness has captured that precious sweet spot where scientific discovery, clinical expertise, compassion, and respect overlap. If you are ready for a journey that may well change your life, then pack this book."

—**Lorimer Moseley, DSc, PhD, FAAHMS, HonFFPMANZFA, HonMAPA**, professor of clinical neuroscience, and director of IIMPACT in Health at the University of South Australia; and CEO of Pain Revolution

"This workbook is a must-have for anyone experiencing chronic pain. Based on science, Rachel Zoffness provides easy-to-follow strategies to understand and change the experience of pain while infusing humor, compassion, authenticity, and courage throughout. Each chapter introduces a new skill, so by the end of the workbook you have everything needed to reclaim your life."

—**Heather Poupore-King, PhD**, clinical assistant professor in the department of anesthesiology and perioperative pain medicine, and director of the Pain Psychology Fellowship at Stanford University School of Medicine

"Rachel Zoffness has done it again. In *The Pain Management Workbook*, she skillfully describes how negative emotions, stress, and anger can impact pain. More importantly, she provides a range of evidence-based, behavioral approaches, including mindfulness, relaxation, and healthy choices—as well as a plethora of exercises to promote transformation. If you are in pain or work with those who are, this workbook contains welcome recipes for self-care and healing."

—**Robert Bonakdar, MD, FAAFP, FACN**, director of pain management at the Scripps Center for Integrative Medicine, coeditor of *Integrative Pain Management*, and 2018 Mayday Pain Advocacy Fellow

"If you feel pain will never end or want alternatives to opioids, *The Pain Management Workbook* provides solutions for taking control of your pain. It's grounded in science, based on extensive clinical experience, and integrates the power of mind and body to mobilize health. The guided practices are actually doable—and promote healing. It's the best self-care workbook that I can recommend."

—**Erik Peper, PhD**, professor of holistic health at San Francisco State University; coauthor of *Tech Stress*; and producer of the blog, peperperspective.com

"Treating chronic pain is one of the most vexing medical challenges that physicians ever confront. In a field offering many approaches to care, Rachel Zoffness's workbook stands out for its comprehensive and scientifically grounded approach to pain management. Her step-by-step, collaborative method promises a clear path toward healing that is realistic and effective. As a physician, I am thrilled to have this valuable tool to recommend to my own patients."

—**Jacob M. Appel, MD, PhD, JD, MPH**, assistant professor of psychiatry and of medical education, and director of ethics education in psychiatry at the Icahn School of Medicine at Mount Sinai

"Rachel Zoffness skillfully unravels the complexities underlying chronic pain, and presents the reader with an approachable way of conceptualizing the condition. She provides a clear, scientifically based pathway to break free from its firm grip and reclaim quality of life. This empowering book is an excellent resource for anyone in pain, or for people wanting to help those living with painful conditions."

—**Ravi Prasad, PhD**, clinical professor and director of behavioral health in the department of anesthesiology and pain medicine at the University of California, Davis School of Medicine

"If you are in chronic pain, want to understand why you have it and what you can do for it, you need not look beyond Rachel Zoffness's excellent book. She has highlighted many of the difficult, important-to-understand concepts of chronic pain, including the biopsychosocial aspects of pain, and offers a mechanism for people to work through their pain."

—**Avinash Ramchandani, MD, MBA, FAAPMR**, board-certified pain management physician specializing in pain medicine at Redwood Pain Institute, part of the Neurovations Group

The

Pain
Management
WORKBOOK

**Powerful CBT and Mindfulness Skills to
Take Control of Pain and Reclaim Your Life**

RACHEL ZOFFNESS, MS, PhD

New Harbinger Publications, Inc.

Publisher's Note

This publication is designed to provide accurate and authoritative information in regard to the subject matter covered. It is sold with the understanding that the publisher is not engaged in rendering psychological, financial, legal, medical, or other professional services. The medical information in this book is provided as an educational resource only, and is not intended to be used or relied upon for any diagnostic or treatment purposes. If expert assistance or counseling is needed, the services of a competent professional should be sought.

Cover design by Amy Shoup

Acquired by Tesilya Hanauer

Edited by Ken Knabb

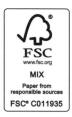

Library of Congress Cataloging-in-Publication Data

Names: Zoffness, Rachel, author.

Title: The pain management workbook : powerful CBT and mindfulness skills to take control of pain and reclaim your life / by Rachel Zoffness, PhD.

Description: Oakland, CA : New Harbinger Publications, [2020] | Includes bibliographical references.

Identifiers: LCCN 2020019883 (print) | LCCN 2020019884 (ebook) | ISBN 9781684036448 (trade paperback) | ISBN 9781684036455 (pdf) | ISBN 9781684036462 (epub)

Subjects: LCSH: Pain--Alternative treatment. | Cognitive therapy. | Mind and body.

Classification: LCC RB127 .Z64 2020 (print) | LCC RB127 (ebook) | DDC 616/.0472--dc23

LC record available at https://lccn.loc.gov/2020019883

LC ebook record available at https://lccn.loc.gov/2020019884

Printed in the United States of America

25   24   23

15   14   13   12   11   10   9   8   7

This book is dedicated to my friend-family, the community that lifts me up and keeps me strong: my most beloved Eisnerites; inspiring UCSF colleagues, collaborators, and co-conspirators; my chronic pain networks; raptorphiles; fellow science nerds, and every other source of support; and every friend who offered a kind word, draft edits, a quiet place to write, a meal, a hike, shelter from the storm, some love, or fuzz therapy…thank you, thank you, thank you.

To every person living with chronic pain: You are not alone. This book is dedicated to you.

Contents

Foreword

For many of us who have apportioned even a small part of our life to the care of others, one inescapable truth is witnessing the difficulty to manage pain. This perspective can be especially challenging when we are faced with our own chronic painful condition or that of a close friend or family member. At the foundation of this experience is the realization that both the mechanisms and personal impact of chronic pain are complex and require a multidimensional approach to restore our physical and emotional well-being. As Professor and Chief of the Division of Pain Medicine at the University of California, San Francisco, I lead an extraordinary team of physicians, scientists, therapists, nurses, and staff who are dedicated to finding ways to restore a person's physical, behavioral, and social health in the setting of chronic pain. It is within this circle of excellence that I have come to know Dr. Rachel Zoffness and to appreciate the critical role she provides in the care and education of patients suffering from chronic pain. Drawing on her extensive clinical experience as a pain psychologist, her deep understanding of evidence-based care, and her role as an educator, she is uniquely qualified to have crafted such a useful and scientifically rigorous manual for adults suffering from chronic painful conditions.

This comprehensive yet approachable workbook is full of practical insights and activities that have the weight of medical research behind them. This should be especially reassuring to anyone suffering, often silently, with chronic pain. Beginning with her first chapter, "Pain Science 101," Dr. Zoffness demystifies chronic pain care by clearly explaining the importance of understanding the *biopsychosocial* model of pain—which indicates that pain has not only biological and neurological components, but also cognitive, emotional, social, and behavioral components. This approach extends throughout the workbook and provides a critical behavioral component to interdisciplinary strategies like physical, pharmacological, and interventional pain medicine techniques. The many strengths of this workbook are drawn from integrating Dr. Zoffness's clinical experience with scientifically proven behavioral techniques that effectively engage the reader. Dr. Zoffness draws us in with examples from everyday life—something that is often lost in classic medical textbooks. Complex neuroscience principles are unwound and presented in intelligible and practical exercises, such as how to control pain volume using our "Pain Dial"; how to avoid cognitive "pain traps" and restore health by challenging our inner "Pain Voice"; how to use "activity pacing" to gradually work one's way back into condition; and many other tactics drawn from cognitive behavioral therapy (CBT) and mindfulness-based stress reduction (MBSR).

In my role overseeing a wide range of approaches to manage chronic pain, behavioral health unquestionably stands as the gatekeeper to long-term recovery. Progress comes not only from expert guidance but also from a narrative of self-directed care and self-compassion. This workbook successfully embraces both aspects of this process. With practical but powerful lifestyle activities, it provides a greatly needed step forward in the integration of behavioral health into pain medicine.

—Mark A. Schumacher, MD, PhD
　　Chief, Division of Pain Medicine,
　　UCSF Department of Anesthesia and Perioperative Care
　　Professor of Anesthesia and Perioperative Care, UCSF

Introduction and Welcome

Welcome! My name is Dr. Rachel Zoffness. I'm a pain psychologist, medical consultant, author, and faculty member at the UCSF School of Medicine, where I teach pain education for medical residents and interns. I was trained in neuroscience, psychology, and human biology at Brown University, Columbia University, St. Luke's–Mt. Sinai Hospital, The Mindful Center, San Diego State University, and the University of California, San Diego. I help people living with pain and medical conditions, and give talks and trainings for healthcare providers around the world.

This workbook is for anyone who's ready to learn how to cope more effectively with pain, as well as for any healthcare provider working with people living with pain. The main goals of this workbook are to:

1. Help you regain control of your brain and body.

2. Reduce pain intensity and frequency.

3. Reduce the impact of pain and illness on your life.

4. Manage triggers so that you have fewer episodes and flare-ups.

5. Teach you to cope more effectively with pain flares once they start.

6. Reduce reliance on pain medications.

7. Improve your quality of life, so you can live a life you love even if you have some pain.

Sometimes people with chronic pain wonder if cognitive behavioral therapy (CBT) or mindfulness has been recommended because they're "crazy" or "it's all in their heads." The answer is *no!* You aren't, and it isn't. Your pain is real. So it can be confusing when a doctor or healthcare provider suggests that you'd benefit from therapy. Here's why this workbook can help: Research shows that medication alone isn't enough. When it comes to pain, "physical" and "emotional" are inextricably intertwined. Each affects the other, all of the time. In order to effectively treat pain, we must therefore target not only biological factors but also cognitive, emotional, behavioral, social, and environmental factors. You'll soon learn about your "pain dial," the pain-control center that lives in your brain and spinal cord and regulates pain volume. This book will give you tools to turn the volume down on pain and regain control of your body. Tools and materials are also available for download at the website for this book: http://www.newharbinger.com/46448. See the back of this book for more details.

Because some people don't understand pain, they can attach stigma and shame to therapy or a workbook like this one. But just as going to the gym to exercise your body doesn't necessarily mean there's something wrong with your body, going to therapy to exercise your mind doesn't necessarily mean there's something wrong with your brain! Rather, it's the opposite: exercising your body makes you stronger and healthier, just as therapy, or brain exercise, makes your mind stronger and healthier. If it's okay to go to a soccer coach to get better at playing soccer, it's certainly okay to use a "pain coach"—such as a CBT therapist, or this workbook!—to help you get better at managing pain.

Pain takes away power. That's just what it does. It makes you feel like your body and your life are no longer under your control. It steals your health, mobility, relationships, sex life, hobbies, job, and dreams. It's time to take that power back. In this book you'll learn all sorts of tips and tools: the purpose of pain, how the brain works, how changing thoughts and emotions can change pain, and important strategies for pain mastery. These skills will give you more control over your body so that pain and illness have less agency over your life. In fact, the more you use this book, the more you'll get out of it. *It only works if you work it.* Think of these strategies as your daily pain medicine: for best results, use them every single day.

Because pharmacological advice is beyond the scope of this book, we'll focus instead on scientifically-supported biobehavioral tools for pain management that have evidence of effectiveness. The exercises in this book are rooted in research, fun to learn, and easy to practice. Some will resonate more than others, so find the activities that are best for you. This knowledge has completely transformed my own chronic pain journey, and I hope it transforms yours, too. I'll be with you every step of the way, rooting for you.

CHAPTER 1

Pain Science 101

If you're struggling with chronic pain, you're not alone. Over one hundred million Americans currently live with chronic pain, and almost all human beings experience pain over the course of their lifetimes. But despite its prevalence, pain is not well understood. Many people living with chronic pain are fed up and frustrated. You may distrust the medical system or feel angry with your healthcare providers. Join the ranks: this is the era of the Opioid Epidemic. The medical system is in the midst of a shakeup and pain treatments are undergoing a revolution.

You might be asking: But how did this happen, and why am I suffering the consequences? Good question. One reason is the fact that, until recently, pain was considered a purely biomedical problem—the result of biological issues like tissue damage and system dysfunction, exclusively. It was therefore believed that pain required purely biomedical solutions, such as medications and surgeries. This has been the predominant approach to pain management for decades. However, while biomedical treatments are important and live-saving, research and clinical evidence indicate that pills and procedures *alone* are insufficient for effectively treating chronic pain. And I'm going to tell you why.

Take a moment to think of three treatments you've tried, as well as their outcome:

1. _____

    Outcome: _____

2. _____

    Outcome: _____

3. _____

    Outcome: _____

While biological processes clearly contribute to pain, science tells us that pain is *not* the result of exclusively biological or medical factors. It's much more complex. Multiple factors influence the pain you feel, including:

Emotions (such as anxiety, depression, hopelessness, and anger);

Cognitive factors (such as thoughts, perceptions, beliefs, and attentional processes);

Environmental context (such as stressors, traumatic experiences, and physical environment); and

Social factors (such as culture, family, socioeconomic status, and access to care).

Indeed, what we now know about pain—and have actually known for decades—is that pain is *biopsychosocial.*

The Three Prongs of Pain: Bio-Psycho-Social

The causes of pain—and therefore the most effective methods for treating it—are biopsychosocial. This means that there are three interconnected, equally important domains to target if we want to effectively treat chronic pain and other health issues: *biology* ("bio"), *psychology* ("psych"), and *social* factors. These three domains overlap to both *produce* and *reduce* pain and symptoms. Because your brain is connected to your body 100% of the time, your social health, emotional health, and physical health are intricately, inextricably intertwined. Let's take a closer look.

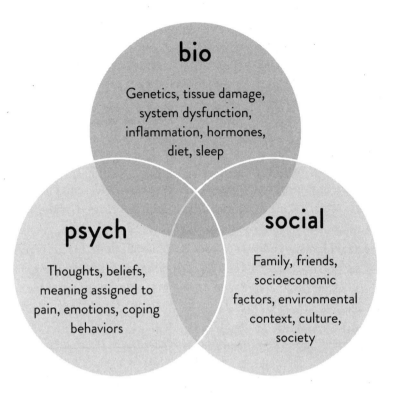

Figure 1: Pain Is Biopsychosocial

Biological components of pain and health include genetics, age, tissue damage, mechanical and anatomical dysfunction, inflammation, immunological issues, and pathology in the pain transmission system. These biological factors are commonly treated with medical interventions such as medications and surgeries. While these interventions are often helpful for acute, or short-term, pain, research suggests they're considerably less helpful for chronic pain. By now you've probably been to many doctor's appointments, had multiple tests and procedures, and tried various medications. Hopefully you have a stellar medical team that has helped you get this far.

Psychological components of health are less commonly addressed, in part because, until recently, we didn't closely link these to physical pain. The psychological domain of pain includes cognitive, emotional, and behavioral factors: emotions, thoughts, beliefs, the *meaning* we assign our pain, memories, prior experiences, expectations, and coping behaviors. Negative thoughts and beliefs that frequently accompany chronic pain, such as "I'll never get better" or "This is hopeless," make us feel worse. Indeed, negative expectations have been shown to amplify pain, resulting in increased signaling from the spinal cord to the brain's pain centers! (We'll cover this in depth in chapters 5 and 6.) Emotions like anxiety, depression, anger, and helplessness also commonly—and understandably—occur when we're sick or in pain. But as you'll soon learn, these negative emotions actually amplify pain. The psychological domain also includes coping behaviors, or how we react in response to pain and illness. Everyone copes with pain differently. Some of us curl up on the couch for days when we hurt. Others push themselves very hard despite the pain and pay a hefty price. The decision to avoid or engage in activities, and how much, has a significant impact on the pain we feel.

The third domain is *social*, or *sociological*. This domain includes cultural, societal, and socioeconomic factors; adverse childhood events like trauma; family factors and relationships; environmental context; and social support. To explain how social factors directly impact pain and health, let's begin with a question: What's the worst punishment you can give a human being? It isn't prison, but good guess. If you misbehave in prison, you're placed in solitary confinement, cut off from all contact and communication with others. What does it say about human beings that the worst thing you can do to us is isolate us?

Humans are social animals, and we evolved to need each other to survive. As you'll learn in the "Social Medicine" section of chapter 7, our brains and bodies release health-promoting chemicals in the presence of others, and health-suppressing stress hormones when we're lonely and isolated. This is supported by research on older adults, which shows higher incidence of pain, disease, depression, disability, and even death among the lonely and isolated. Indeed, being isolated at home, missing work and social activities, and stopping hobbies can actually make pain worse. As you'll soon learn, the opposite is also true: when you improve social functioning, you can also reduce your *pain*. Social components of pain additionally include socioeconomic, cultural, and environmental factors like culture, race, income, unemployment, access to healthcare, inadequate housing, abuse, and trauma.

Not surprisingly, these three domains are all interconnected:

- *Social* factors affect hormones and brain chemistry (*biology*) as well as thoughts and emotions (*psychology*);

- Changes in emotions like stress and anxiety (*psychology*) alter brain chemistry, hormone levels, and immune functioning (*biology*);

- Tending to sleep and nutritional needs (*biology*) can improve mood (*psychology*) and social functioning.

Everything is intertwined. Taking care of one domain affects all domains. This is because your brain and body are inextricably interconnected.

When it comes to pain, dividing humans into two disconnected entities—mind ("mental") and body ("physical")—couldn't be less helpful or more wrong. Indeed, an exclusive focus on the "bio" domain of pain *misses two-thirds of the pain problem!*

Pain = Biology + Psychology + Social Factors

What biological, psychological, and sociological factors do you suspect contribute to your pain?

Biological: _____

_____

Psychological: _____

_____

Social, cultural, or environmental: _____

_____

The biopsychosocial approach to pain management is the basis of this workbook. Welcome, I'm honored to have you here! You're about to take the reins, harness your brain's power, and change your pain.

The Power of Pain Education

Before we delve into managing pain, it's critical to first understand your pain from the inside out. There's real power in understanding pain. In fact, research suggests that *understanding* your pain can actually *change* your pain, particularly when combined with pain-management tools like the ones in this book. How is this possible?

Pain commonly brings with it fear, anxiety, and dread. As you'll soon learn, these are the very emotions that perpetuate the chronic pain cycle, leading to the maintenance and exacerbation of pain. However, when people understand their pain—how it works, what it signals and what it doesn't, what makes it worse, and what factors help—the cycle can be interrupted. Pain education can result in increased hope and motivation, reduced catastrophic thinking, more accurate perceptions of pain, less fear of movement, decreased disability, improved physical performance, fewer doctor's appointments and medical procedures, and less pain! So let's begin at the beginning and start your healing journey by learning more about pain.

What Is Pain?

The question I get asked most is: "Do you treat physical pain or emotional pain?" My answer is always: "Yes." The International Association for the Study of Pain defines pain as "an unpleasant sensory and emotional experience." According to the experts, pain is both physical *and* emotional, 100% of the time. It's never just one or the other.

$$Pain = Physical + Emotional$$

Indeed, neuroscience shows that pain is what we call a "diffuse neurological process." That is, there is no one, single "pain center" in the brain responsible for producing the experience of pain. Instead, there are multiple brain sites that contribute. These include the parts of your brain responsible for:

Thoughts (cerebral cortex),

Emotions (limbic system), and

Attentional processes (prefrontal cortex).

Other regions of the brain implicated in pain production include the thalamus (the brain's relay station); the anterior cingulate cortex (registers the "emotional unpleasantness" of pain); the insular cortex (encodes pain intensity, links sensory input with emotion); the somatosensory cortex (processes sensory information from the body, including the location of pain); primary motor cortex (involved in movement away from painful stimuli); the hippocampus (stores "pain memories" from as far back as childhood); and the amygdala (locus of fear, anxiety, and other emotions).

Your brain then puts all of this together, integrating cognitive, emotional, sensory, and other information to generate and regulate pain. This means that how you *think* and how you *feel* affect your experience of pain. And not just some of the time, but *all* of the time. Consider the words used to describe pain. For example, I describe my chronic leg pain as burning, shooting, miserable, and frustrating.

What words describe your pain?

_____

_____

Did you use both physical and emotional words in your description, like I did? That's because pain isn't just physical—it's also emotional!

Acute versus Chronic Pain

Pain is a complex subjective experience that comes in all shapes and sizes. If you feel it, it's real—and no one should ever tell you otherwise. Some pain comes and goes quickly, vanishing within three months. This is called *acute*, or short-term, pain, and is typically the result of an injury or acute illness. A broken bone, second-degree burn, the pain of childbirth, or muscle pain from the flu are all examples of acute pain. Other pain is more stubborn and enduring. If pain persists beyond the expected healing time, it's called *chronic* or *persistent pain*—typically defined as pain lasting three months or longer. Chronic pain can be linked to a condition—migraine, fibromyalgia, sickle cell disease, cancer—or it may have no known cause. Both acute and chronic pain can be experienced anywhere in your body: head, back, stomach, elbow.

What condition or conditions are you coping with, and where do you hurt?

_____

_____

_____

For how long have you been in pain?

_____

Why Do We Have Pain?

It may sound wonderful to never have pain—it certainly does to me. However, pain evolved and endures in humans because it can be a life-saving mechanism. In fact, individuals born without the ability to feel pain don't live very long. Why? Because pain is your body's *warning system*, built to respond to potential danger and alert you to threats to safety and well-being. In fact, if pain weren't horrible, it wouldn't get your attention—and that's pain's job. Pain that isn't bothersome fails to change your behavior enough to protect you.

Your pain warning system tells you when you've stepped on a nail and need to pull it out, to run from a hive of wasps after you get stung, and to stop and rest after a head injury. By giving you unpleasant feelings, pain buys you time to heal and teaches you to avoid dangerous situations in the future. Believe it or not, pain is generally a good thing. It's your body's way of keeping you safe and alive. In fact, pain is essential for survival.

Name two instances in which pain served to help and protect you (*for example, muscle soreness after a workout; pain after burning your hand on a hot pan*):

1. _____

2. _____

How Pain Works

It's easy to believe that pain is exclusively located in the body, in the place that hurts. But despite the fact that we experience pain in our bodies, pain is actually constructed by the *brain*.

Evidence of the brain's role in pain comes from a medical phenomenon known as phantom limb pain. This condition arises when an accident survivor loses a limb, then continues to feel terrible pain in the missing limb even after it's gone. If pain was located exclusively in the body, *no limb should mean no pain!* Pain, then, must be constructed elsewhere, and science tells us that it is constructed by the brain.

Your amazing brain is part of your *central nervous system* (CNS), made up of your brain and spinal cord. The CNS is the command center of your body, in charge of major bodily functions like movement and thought. There is always two-way traffic in the spinal cord sending information up from body to brain, and back down from brain to body. These ascending (body to brain) and descending (brain to body) messages constantly regulate your experience of pain, along with a host of immunological, hormonal, muscular, and chemical changes in the body.

The basic functioning of your pain system starts with sensory receptors in your body called *nociceptors,* which collect information from the world around you and alert you to potentially damaging stimuli by detecting extremes in temperature, pressure, and chemicals. You have multiple types of nociceptors, including thermoreceptors (sensitive to temperature extremes); mechanoreceptors (stimulated by changes in pressure, tension, or movement); and chemoreceptors (stimulated by potentially dangerous chemicals). Information from these sensory receptors travels up your spinal cord to your brain. Your brain then interprets these signals and decides how to respond: Is there an emergency, or is this a false alarm? What behaviors need to change in order for you to stay protected and safe?

If there's any reason to think that protection is required, *your brain makes pain.* Your appraisal of the situation is a critical determinant of the pain you feel. Context, thoughts, prior experiences and memories, emotions, and the meaning you assign to your pain all change your experience of it. Put another way, *pain is not an accurate indicator of tissue damage.* Pain is an interpretation, your brain's best guesstimate based on all available information.

Of course, pain often does indicate that the body is in danger. Let's say, for example, you trip on a concrete sidewalk while running and break your ankle. Sensory receptors in your body send *warning messages* from your ankle up to your spinal cord, where motor neurons initiate movements that quickly change your behavior so that you can protect yourself. This process is called *nociception,* and nearly all animals, even those with simple nervous systems, experience it.

There is also the conscious recognition of potential harm, which is communicated via sensory signals from the body, through the spinal cord, and up to the brain, alerting you of possible danger. This information is shared with various parts of the brain, including your emotion center, which all work together to reach a conclusion about how to respond. Some of the information the brain incorporates is context (fell on concrete!), past experiences (similar fall last year!), prior knowledge (possible injury!), emotions (panic!), and physiological responses (bruising, swelling).

The brain then sends messages back down to your body via the spinal cord, saying: *"Danger! PAIN! Yeeeouch, stop running!"* This conscious pain response further informs subsequent decisions and actions, stopping you in your tracks and changing your behavior to prevent further damage to bone and tissue. Imagine what would happen if you just kept going…? It may sound wonderful to never feel pain, but without it you'd have seriously damaged your leg on that run, because you wouldn't have been motivated to stop.

Describe a time your pain alarm helpfully warned you to change your behavior, protecting you from harm. What did you *do* in response to pain?

_____

_____

The pain system, like most systems, is imperfect. Sometimes there are glitches. For example, the brain can misinterpret a warning signal from the body as "dangerous" even in the absence of true danger, resulting in the generation or amplification of pain for weeks and months when no protection is actually required. When this happens, pain really gets to be a pain. Chronic, ongoing pain can interrupt your life, compel you to quit work and hobbies, prevent you from spending quality time with family and friends, terminate your sex life, and even prevent you from leaving the house. It can make you feel angry, depressed, anxious, and afraid.

What activities has your pain stopped you from doing?

1. _____

2. _____

3. _____

Context Matters

Because pain is a guesstimate—your brain's best assessment of whether your body requires protection, and how much—*context* is critically important. Context is the sum total of all available information from your internal and external environments. Context includes—but isn't limited to—information from your five senses, including where you are, whom you are with, and what's happening; past experiences and memories; thoughts, beliefs, and expectations; emotions; future predictions, and prior knowledge.

For example, an arm pinch feels worse if made by a frighteningly long needle than by a friend's loving, reassuring squeeze. Unexpected leg pain on an airplane hurts more if you believe it's due to a lethal blood clot than if you think it's from sitting for too long. If you injure yourself at work on a stressful day, that very same injury can feel worse than if acquired on a pleasant, relaxing Sunday afternoon. Memories of a previous painful concussion can exacerbate the pain of a new and different head injury. Pain feels worse when you're lonely and sad than when you're happy and surrounded by people you love. Pleasant colors and soothing surroundings can make pain feel less bad, which is why children's hospitals are often festooned with colorful murals and stuffed animals. If you take a sugar pill—a placebo—*believing* that it's an effective pain medication, your pain may subside simply because you believe it will. In summary: *indications of danger make pain worse, while credible evidence of safety reduces pain.*

Name a time you noticed that context influenced your pain: _____

_____

This important premise is effectively demonstrated by two clinical cases from pain research, which I call "A Tale of Two Nails."

Case 1: A construction worker jumped off a plank at a construction site straight onto a seven-inch nail, which penetrated his boot clear through to the other side. His pain was so severe that he was rushed to the hospital and sedated with pain medication. When the doctors removed his boot, they discovered a miracle: the nail had passed through the space *between* his toes, without ever penetrating his skin. Despite initial appearances, there was no damage to the man's foot—no blood, no puncture wound, not even a scratch. But make no mistake: despite the absence of tissue damage, his pain was real. So what happened?

The man's sensory receptors—his "danger detectors"—reported to his brain that there'd been an accident, that a nail had penetrated his boot. His brain, perceiving potential threat to his safety and well-being, used context to determine what had occurred, collecting information from his five senses (including the visual of a nail sticking out of his shoe!), knowledge of the dangerous work environment and its risks, his coworkers' horrified faces, and other data to make a guesstimate about what had happened and how to respond. Thoughts, beliefs, and emotions, including panic and fear, set off a cascade of biological and neurochemical processes. His brain, synthesizing the sum total of this information, decided that he was in danger, so *it made pain to protect him.* In this case, real pain was generated entirely as a result of factors having nothing to do with actual tissue damage—yet was as intense as if he'd been stabbed.

Case 2: Another construction worker (dangerous job, that!) was using a nail gun on a job site when it unexpectedly backfired, clocking him in the face. Other than a mild toothache and a bruise under his jaw, he thought he'd escaped unscathed, so went about his business. Six days later—six days of eating, sleeping, and going to work—he went to the dentist. Much to his surprise, an X-ray revealed a four-inch nail embedded in his head! Because contextual cues failed to put his brain on high alert, his pain system remained relatively quiet—despite actual bodily harm and need for serious medical intervention.

These Tales of Two Nails highlight a number of important points (pun intended!) for pain sufferers and healthcare providers. The first is that *pain is not an accurate indicator of tissue damage*. You can experience terrible pain in the complete absence of bodily harm (such as a nail in the shoe but not the foot), and little pain in the presence of significant damage (such as a nail to the face!). That is: just because something hurts does not necessarily mean your body is in danger of harm. *"Hurt" and "harm" are not the same.*

The second takeaway is that thoughts, perceptions, emotions, context, and the meaning you assign pain—in addition to sensory inputs from the body—define the human experience of pain, both amplifying and reducing it. You've likely experienced this phenomenon many times. For example, have you ever played a soccer game that was so much fun you didn't realize your leg was bleeding until after the game was over? Or discovered mysterious black-and-blue marks in the shower, having no idea how they got there?

If so, record here:

_____

_____

Athletes regularly report discovering blood and bruises only after the game is over, even though the injury occurred hours before. Indeed, cognitive, emotional, and contextual factors like excitement, distraction, pleasure, perception of safety, and lack of conscious awareness can keep pain at bay. This exemplifies an important, and counterintuitive, point: *Injury can occur in the absence of pain, and pain can occur in the absence of injury.*

This disconnect between "pain" and "damage" has also been historically reported during wartime, when physicians noticed that the extent of soldiers' injuries didn't correlate with the degree of pain they experienced. This specifically applied to soldiers safely off the battlefield, soothed with news they were out of harm's way and would soon be going home. Similarly, studies on back pain reveal that there's little to no correlation between back scan "abnormalities" and pain. In one study, disk degeneration and bulges were found in 80% of elderly patients who had *no symptoms or pain*. In another, MRI "abnormalities" were found to be completely unrelated to the degree of disability or pain intensity reported by patients: some people with lumps and bumps had pain, and others with similar back scans had none. Scientists have therefore concluded that, like the wrinkles on our faces, "wrinkles" on our spines are likely a normal part of aging. However, these back scan results are often incorrectly blamed as the sole cause of pain—leading to unnecessary surgeries and medical interventions, often without relief. This has resulted in the addition of another diagnosis to the medical literature: Failed Back Surgery Syndrome. Indeed, up to 40% of back surgeries are unsuccessful, suggesting that surgery may not be the cure for back pain. Like every other type of pain, the cause of, and most effective treatment for, back pain is *biopsychosocial*.

Your Pain System Is "Plastic"

While it's easy to believe that chronic pain will never lessen or change, there's evidence to suggest that this isn't true. Neuroscience tells us that your brain's pain centers are *not* "hardwired," that is, the connections between brain cells are *not* fixed nor permanent, and your brain isn't doomed to remain the same simply because of genetic makeup or medical condition. Rather, experiences, environment, and other inputs constantly shape the structure and function of your pain system.

Nerve cells in the brain, called *neurons*, have the ability to change and reorganize over time. Neurons grow, shrink, move, and form entirely new networks depending on input and experience, compensating for injury and disease and adjusting their activities in response to environmental changes and new situations. Brain activity associated with a particular function, like sight, can be transferred to a different brain location; brain volume in specific sites—like the part of your brain responsible for memory—can increase or decrease; and *synapses*, or connections between brain cells, can strengthen and weaken over time. There can be microscopic changes in individual neurons, and there can be large-scale changes to the overall map of your brain.

The term we use to describe the brain's remarkable ability to grow and change is *neuroplasticity*—"plastic" meaning that the brain ("neuro") is flexible and malleable, the opposite of fixed and permanent. Similarly, your body's biological systems are also "plastic" and can adapt and change over time, like the way your muscles grow with use and shrink with disuse.

Your wonderfully plastic brain is constantly changing and morphing to suit your needs and your environment. Every time you learn something new—a foreign language, how to drive stick shift, Aunt Mary's secret sausage recipe—your brain changes. The more you practice this new skill, the bigger and stronger the brain pathways dedicated to that skill become. This phenomenon is known as "Neurons that fire together, wire together."

Similarly, every time you forget something—a math formula, a colleague's name, a regrettable event from college days (perhaps it would be better if we forgot more of those?)—your brain also changes. Forgetting is the result of expendable neural pathways that are pruned, just as you'd trim dead branches from a tree. This phenomenon is called "Use it or lose it."

. . . But how does this apply to pain?

Chronic Pain Changes the Brain

Your brain is *amazing* at learning. If you want to become good at something—playing chess, cooking flambé, drawing maps—just practice it over and over and your brain will get better at it. Just as your bicep muscles get bigger and stronger with use, frequently used brain pathways also get bigger and stronger with use. This neuroplastic change occurs because, as you now know, "neurons that fire together, wire together."

To demonstrate how this works, consider this: many years ago I wanted to be a superb piano player. After months of practice, it was as if my fingers knew the songs. I didn't need to think—my fingers just played the music. A change had occurred in the parts of my brain coding for sound, memory, and motor coordination. How did this happen? Well, the more I practiced, the more I used the "piano pathway" in my brain. The more I used this "piano pathway," the bigger and stronger it got, and the better I became at playing.

Your brain has also successfully learned many things. What are some skills you've practiced and gotten good at over time?

1. _____

2. _____

3. _____

Just as the brain can become good at piano playing, map drawing, and flambé making, it can also become really good at *pain*. When you have pain for weeks, months, and years, your brain inadvertently "practices" pain.

The longer you practice pain, the more you use the "pain pathway" in your brain. The more you use this pathway, the bigger and stronger it gets. The stronger this pathway gets, the better your brain gets at pain! When this happens, we say your brain has become *sensitive*. Your central nervous system (CNS: your brain + spinal cord) and peripheral nervous system (PNS: the rest of your body) can both become sensitive.

Chronic Pain Is a False Alarm

When your brain is *sensitive*, it has a lower threshold for sensory stimuli. For example, if you have a sensitive sense of smell, you detect faint scents that other people hardly notice, so they seem magnified and you pick up on them more. Some animals, like dogs, are sensitive to sound—they detect sounds humans can't even hear. And sounds that seem loud to us are even louder to dogs: across America, dogs whimper under beds during Independence Day fireworks.

Similarly, people with chronic pain can become sensitive to *warning messages* from the body. To you, these messages seem magnified and your brain picks up on them more. When your pain pathway has gotten big and strong, we say that pain volume is now very "loud." Small signals from your body now sound—and feel—huge, so warning messages are interpreted as signs of danger even when your body is safe. In other words, your warning system has become highly reactive.

As with any alarm system, there can be false alarms. With chronic pain, your body's warning system "goes off" even when nothing's wrong—like when your car alarm goes off even though there's no break-in. Sometimes the brain sounds the pain alarm when in truth, despite your *very real* pain and discomfort, you're not actually in danger.

This is in part due to your brain's prefrontal cortex, which is responsible for regulating attentional processes. Once the brain is sensitized and hyper-attuned to possible danger, it chronically scans the environment for threats, sometimes finding some where there are none. Your entire "danger-detection" system is now on high alert—but it doesn't need to be. In fact, this constant attention to, and focus on, pain *only makes pain worse*. These warning signals are therefore no longer useful, nor do they protect you. Your nervous system has simply "gotten good" at pain, so your brain's response is louder.

Hurt and Harm Are Not the Same

It's easy to believe that if something *hurts*, it's *harming* your body. Indeed, the pain system exists to warn us of threats to safety. But pain is not always an indicator of danger, or harm.

Let's define our terms:

Hurt: the uncomfortable sensation of pain; for example, the hurt you feel after stubbing your toe.

Harm: physical damage to your body; for example, the purple bruise and swelling left behind by that stub, evidence of crushed capillaries and inflammation.

When you have acute, short-term pain, "hurt" is often an important indicator of damage or potential danger. Take, for example, that broken ankle sustained on your run: If you try to keep running, your brain will respond with a strong warning message that says, *Stop!* This pain grabs your attention and tells you to sit and rest—because if you run on a broken ankle, you'll further damage the bones, muscle, and tissue in your leg, and significantly harm your body.

However, when pain becomes chronic, it's an unreliable indicator of danger or harm. Instead, you experience a false alarm that leads you to believe you're in danger—even when you're not. When you sense danger, your body responds with stress and fear. As you'll soon learn, stress and fear further sensitize your pain system, making pain even worse.

For these reasons, it's important to understand that, when you have chronic pain, *the pain you feel isn't necessarily a signal that you're in danger of harm.* While the pain is real, the danger is not! For example:

- Going for a walk when you have daily migraines might hurt, but it isn't going to harm your head.

- Having a picnic in the park when you have fibromyalgia might hurt, but it will not harm your body.

- Riding a stationary bike when you're fatigued and achy from Lyme disease might make you feel tired, but it isn't harmful.

In fact, the opposite is true: movement and exercise help retrain your pain system, ultimately turning the volume down on those unnecessarily loud signals.

Before you can turn off this false alarm, you must first understand when you're at risk of actual harm—like a stomachache after eating shellfish, warning you of a dangerous allergic reaction—and when you're *not* at risk of harm, like while walking during recovery from complex regional pain syndrome (CRPS) and noticing pain in the affected foot. For many painful conditions and illnesses, pain is *not* necessarily a signal that your body is being harmed.

Can you think of a time you hurt, but your body wasn't in danger of damage or harm?

_____

_____

_____

Neuroplasticity: Retraining Your Pain System

The good news is this: because your brain and body are plastic, you can start retraining your pain system right away. Today! One way to help your sensitive nervous system is to *desensitize* it. When you desensitize brain and body, you reduce your level of pain sensitivity, decrease pain-related fear, and turn the volume down on pain.

The best way to do this is via *gradual exposure* to small doses of potentially triggering stimuli such as movement, touch, and activity. The process of desensitization may sound complicated, but in reality your brain and body desensitize to stimuli all the time. For example, have you ever walked into a room that reeked of trash, only to stop noticing the odor a few minutes later? Hey presto: your brain became desensitized to the scent.

In this book, you'll learn techniques to desensitize brain and body and control your pain. By teaching the brain that not all pain is dangerous—that *hurt and harm are not the same*—you'll encourage the creation of new brain pathways associating activity and movement with *safety* instead of danger. You'll learn how to gradually expose your sensitized pain system to small doses of activity and stimuli that initially get a big pain reaction, like walking with back pain or socializing with fibromyalgia, so that over time the pain response gets lower…and lower…and lower…until your brain eventually just stops alarm-ing.

It may sound impossible—but you, too, can create an "off" button for your brain's pain alarm. By pushing this off button repeatedly—multiple times a day every day—using the exercises in this book, you'll weaken the association between "pain" and "danger," pruning that faulty neural pathway. Over time, as you slowly get used to small amounts of activity and stimulation, your brain will learn that "hurt" doesn't necessarily mean "danger" or "harm." This will help your nervous system rewire, turning the volume down on those big warning signals so that they're smaller and less loud.

Desensitization is a critical part of breaking the pain cycle.

An important way to accomplish this is by doing things: going outside, moving your body, seeing friends, and stimulating your powerful and amazing brain! It sounds counterintuitive, I know. When you have pain, it's normal to believe you're supposed to stay home and rest. That's what most of us do in response to pain and illness. And it's true that you need short-term rest to recover from a procedure, sickness, or acute injury.

But staying home and not moving when you have chronic, long-term pain is a *trap*. Being sedentary and missing out on life for long stretches of time makes pain worse because your nervous system stays sensitized to, and focused on, the pain. The false-alarm system keeps shrieking loudly with nothing to control its volume. In fact, the longer you stay home avoiding activity, the longer your brain will stay in this sensitive, protective state, and the longer your pain will last. It happens to many of us: when my chronic pain developed, I lay on my couch "recovering" for more than a year.

What's the longest you've stayed home or inside?

_____

Before learning to retrain your pain system—and you will!—you first need to know how thoughts and feelings affect pain.

An Introduction to Your Pain Dial

The pain system is complicated. To help you understand it, here's an analogy: Imagine you have a *pain dial* in your CNS that controls pain volume, similar to the volume knob on your car stereo. The function of this dial is to protect you from harm. Any time your brain perceives or believes that your body is in danger, the pain dial is turned up, so pain volume is loud—loud enough to grab your attention, change your behavior, and get you out of harm's way. However, if your brain determines that your body is safe, the dial is turned down—so pain volume is lower, and warning signals are quieter.

Actual or perceived danger = Pain volume up

Actual or perceived safety = Pain volume down

Your pain dial can also be adjusted by:

1.   Stress and anxiety,

2.   Mood, and

3.   Attention.

Specifically, when you're feeling *stressed and anxious*—

your body is tense and tight,

you're having worried thoughts, and

you perceive or believe your body is in danger—

your cerebral cortex and limbic system (which control thoughts and feelings) send signals to your pain dial, turning it way up.

Your brain, interpreting this as an emergency, generates loud signals that sound like this:

PAIN!!!!!!!!!! PAIN!!!!!!!!!!

PAAAAAAIIIIIINNNN!!!!!!!!!!!!!!!

The pain dial is also controlled by negative emotions like sadness, anger, hopelessness, and frustration.

When your *mood* is low and thoughts are negative,

your brain amplifies danger messages

so that pain volume is pushed up,

making pain worse.

This is also true when *attention* is focused on pain.

When you're home in bed,

missing work and social events,

and focused on your pain,

> your prefrontal cortex (which controls attention) sends signals to your pain dial,
>
> turning it way up,
>
> making pain worse.

But have no fear…the opposite is also true!

When *stress and anxiety* are low—

your body is relaxed,

your thoughts are calm,

you perceive or believe that your body is safe—

> your cerebral cortex and limbic system send signals to your pain dial,
>
> lowering the volume on pain,
>
> so that pain feels less bad.

And when your *mood* is high—

you're engaged in pleasurable activities,

your thoughts are positive,

and you're feeling happy—

> your brain determines that little protection is needed,
>
> so pain volume is reduced.

And finally, when you're *distracted*—

your attention is focused on things other than pain, like social activities, watching funny movies with friends and stuffing your face with popcorn—

> the pain dial is turned down,
>
> so pain feels less bad.

This means that when you're *relaxed, happy, distracted, and believe your body is safe*, pain is quieter. Signals sound like this:

PAIN. PAIN.

PAIN.

The pain is still there—it hasn't magically disappeared—but it *feels less bad*.

The conclusion of this analogy is thus: *Thoughts, beliefs, emotions, perceptions, coping behaviors, and context can adjust pain volume.*

It worked this way for Ethan.

Ethan's Story

Ethan, seventy-two years old and living alone, had recently undergone knee-replacement surgery. His daily pain was ten out of ten. He was wheelchair-bound for months, unable to participate in activities or self-care, worried he'd never walk again. One day his granddaughter came to visit and brought friends. They sat together on the couch looking through Ethan's old photo albums, telling stories and giggling. His granddaughter baked warm cookies. Ethan was so engrossed in reminiscing—enjoying the stories, cookies, and company—that he "forgot" about his pain. It wasn't until his granddaughter left that Ethan realized he'd forgotten to take his afternoon dose of pain medication. The combination of relaxation, laughter, company, pleasure, *and* distraction *was like a magic medicine that turned down his pain dial without him even realizing it.*

Describe a time when you were distracted, happy, relaxed, or having fun, and briefly "forgot" your pain or it felt a little less bad:

_____

_____

If thoughts, beliefs, and emotions can amplify and reduce pain, this means that you have more control over your pain than you may have realized! In fact, *you can take control of your pain dial* by managing *(1) stress and anxiety, (2) mood, (3) attention, (4) interpretations and understanding of pain,* and *(5) coping behaviors.*

To manage expectations, it's also important to clarify what this does *not* mean. Regulating emotional, behavioral, cognitive, and contextual factors is not an instant, magical cure for pain. While these strategies can be very powerful, "up" and "down" on the pain dial aren't necessarily the same as "on" and "off." You're not going to instantly or permanently feel better, never to have pain again, just because you're briefly happy and distracted. No false promises here. That said, research shows that effective pain control requires a rewiring of the pain system via a biopsychosocial approach, targeting cognitive, emotional, behavioral, and environmental inputs. This necessitates creating and strengthening new brain pathways while weakening old ones. This can be done by practicing the pain-management skills in this book over and over and over again. Try using them every day, repeatedly pushing the "off" button on your pain alarm until it becomes automatic. Remember: neurons that fire, wire! The more you practice pain control, the bigger and stronger your "pain-control pathway" will get.

Download this "Pain Dial Review" at http://www.newharbinger.com/46448. Put a copy on your fridge, tape one next to your bed, and bring one to work.

PAIN DIAL REVIEW

Volume high = Pain feels worse
Perception or belief that your body is in danger
Stressed or anxious
Body tense and tight
Worried thoughts
Negative mood
Attention focused on pain
Staying inside or in bed for long periods

Volume low = Pain feels less bad
Perception or belief that your body is safe
Relaxed
Body loose and less stressed
Calm thoughts
Positive mood
Distracted, attention focused elsewhere
Going outside, moving, and engaging in activities

Lower Your Pain Volume

To begin taking power back from pain, brainstorm activities that improve your mood, relax your body and mind, and distract you. These will help reduce pain volume. In order to heal, your nervous system needs exposure to sunlight, real-world activities, and people, so try to choose activities that don't center exclusively on screens. See Ellie's example:

What lifts your mood?

Ellie's list:

1. My Saturday dance class

2. Watching my cat try to figure out the dripping faucet

3. Reading cooking blogs

4. Raspberry chocolate chip ice cream

Your list:

1. _____

2. _____

3. _____

4. _____

What relaxes your body?

Ellie's list:

1. A hot bath

2. Going for nature walks

3. Getting a back massage

4. Stretching and yoga

Your list:

1. _____

2. _____

3. _____

4. _____

What relaxes your mind?

Ellie's list:

1. Telling myself that everything is going to be okay

2. Imagining I'm on my favorite beach in Mexico

3. Listening to thunderstorms on a relaxation app

4. Practicing mindfulness

Your list:

1. _____

2. _____

3. _____

4. _____

What distracts you?

Ellie's list:

1. Crossword puzzles and brainteasers

2. Complicated chicken recipes

3. Painting with watercolors

4. Counting backward from two hundred by seven

Your list:

1. _____

2. _____

3. _____

4. _____

Pain Dial Worksheet

List five things that *raise* your pain volume and make pain worse. Include activities and beliefs that signal danger, make you feel stressed or worried, trigger negative emotions like sadness or anger, and focus attention on pain instead of away from it. See Simon's example.

Simon's list:

1. When people ask about my pain (increased attention on pain)

2. Doing nothing at home, especially when my wife and kids are enjoying activities together without me (high stress, low mood, increased attention)

3. A pile of work that feels too big to finish (high stress)

4. Believing that leg pain means I'll never walk again (belief that my body is in danger, high stress, low mood)

5. When I stop playing pickup basketball on weekends because I'm in pain (low mood, increased attention)

Your list:

1. _____

2. _____

3. _____

4. _____

5. _____

Now list five things that *lower* your pain volume. Include ideas from the "Lower Your Pain Volume" activity that make you feel safe, lift your mood, help you feel relaxed and calm, and distract you from pain.

Simon's list:

Five things that lower my pain volume:

1. Reading a good book (relaxed, good mood, distracted)

2. Going for a walk in the sunshine and petting dogs (relaxed, good mood, distracted)

3. Dinner at an Italian restaurant with friends (relaxed, good mood, distracted)

4. Watching basketball games with my son (relaxed, good mood, distracted)

5. Reminding myself that hurt doesn't equal harm (belief that my body is safe, relaxed)

Your list:

1. _____

2. _____

3. _____

4. _____

5. _____

Conclusion

Pain is biopsychosocial—both physical *and* emotional—and is informed by bodily sensations, context, interpretations, thoughts, and emotions. Constructed by brain and body working in concert, pain serves as your warning system, motivating you to change your behavior in response to perceived danger. Because pain is not an accurate indicator of tissue damage, it's important to notice the meaning you assign your pain, and to distinguish "hurt" from "harm."

Once you realize that pain isn't always a sign of damage and may instead be a false alarm, you can start taking steps to get your life back. This is best done using medical interventions *plus* psychosocial strategies to target thoughts, beliefs, emotions, coping behaviors, social functioning, and environmental context. Effective tools to retrain your nervous system, change your plastic brain, and turn down your pain dial can be found throughout this book. You'll learn skills from cognitive behavioral therapy (CBT), mindfulness-based stress reduction (MBSR), and other evidence-based approaches to help you gain power over pain and illness. These strategies can help you resume your life and get back to doing the things you love! We'll start by learning more about the inextricable link between "physical" and "emotional."

CHAPTER 2

CBT Basics: Triggers, Emotions, and Coping with Pain

Many of us have been taught that mind and body, mental and physical, are two separate entities, to be treated independently. This simply isn't true. Mind and body are *always* connected, each constantly affecting the other. This fact is particularly important when it comes to understanding pain. Pain is the result of mind and body working together, including your limbic system—the brain's "emotion center."

The Inextricable Link Between Physical and Emotional

It may seem illogical that your emotional state should impact how good or bad your back, leg, or head feel on any given day. But there's just no denying it: emotions affect pain. Research shows that negative emotions like stress, anger, and sadness amplify pain, while positive emotions like relaxation, joy, and happiness can reduce pain. This means that pain is never just physical, it's also emotional! Therefore, in order to effectively treat pain, we must address thoughts and feelings in addition to physical symptoms.

One scientifically-supported treatment for chronic pain is *cognitive behavioral therapy* (CBT). In concert with medical treatment, this intervention can target all three biopsychosocial domains. CBT has evidence of effectiveness for chronic pain and illness, sleep, anxiety, depression, family conflict, and other issues commonly associated with chronic pain. Studies suggest that CBT can change brain and behavior to facilitate improved functioning and quality of life; reduce reliance on pain medication; decrease the stress, anxiety, and sadness associated with chronic pain; and even lower the pain dial to decrease pain itself.

Because some people don't understand pain, they may attach stigma and shame to therapy or to a workbook like this one. But just as going to the gym to exercise your body doesn't necessarily mean there's something wrong with your body, going to therapy to exercise your mind doesn't necessarily mean there's something wrong with your brain! Rather, it's the opposite: exercising your body makes you stronger and healthier, just as therapy, or brain exercise, makes you stronger and healthier. Just as a soccer coach can help you get better at soccer, a "pain coach," such as a CBT therapist—or this workbook!—can help you get better at living with pain.

Coping with chronic pain is hard. It's naturally associated with feelings of anxiety, fear, depressed mood, and hopelessness. Having these emotions does not mean you're "mentally ill." Rather, these are normal reactions to an abnormal situation: your body simply wasn't built to endure pain month after month, year after year. CBT can therefore target the thoughts, beliefs, emotions, and coping behaviors that keep your pain cycle cycling and keep your life on hold. If you find a therapist covered by your insurance who hasn't been trained in pain management, hand him or her this workbook—it contains an entire CBT-for-pain protocol. You need not go it alone! And you deserve support.

An Introduction to CBT

To effectively treat chronic pain, we must target biology, psychology, and sociological factors, including social functioning. These interconnected elements are central to CBT, which teaches us that:

- what we *think*

- affects how we *feel emotionally*

- affects how we *feel physically*

- affects how we *act* (or behave)

… 'round and 'round in a circle, each affecting the others. These four components—thoughts, emotions, sensations, and behaviors—interact to affect pain. This process is outlined in the *CBT Pain Cycle*, below.

The CBT cycle starts with a *trigger*, which is a difficult situation or event. Triggers can be anything from a pain flare, to a scary test result, to an argument with family. Triggering events then generate thoughts, feelings, bodily sensations, and behaviors, which all affect one another. For this example, our trigger will be pain.

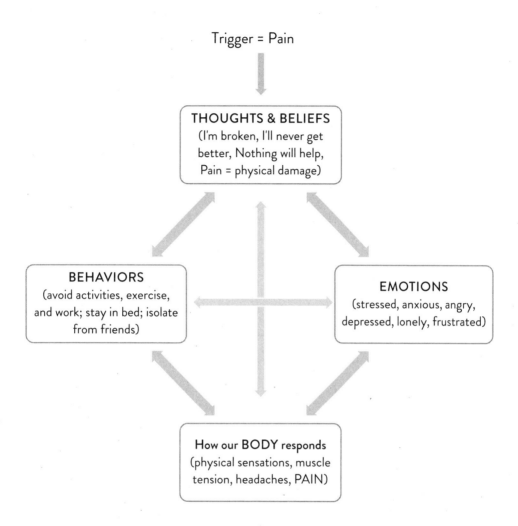

Figure 2: CBT Pain Cycle

Say you have a pain flare that prevents you from going to work on an important day or that cancels your plans. The next thing that happens is that your brain thinks a thought. These thoughts typically happen so quickly that we call them "*automatic.*" Similar to the process of blinking, you think—and blink—thousands of times a day, but not always consciously. With pain or illness, automatic thoughts are often, and understandably, negative. Some common automatic negative thoughts that occur when we have pain are: "Nothing can help me," and "My life is miserable. I can't deal with this." Negative thoughts can have a major impact on pain and health. You'll see how in chapter 5.

Negative Emotions Amplify Pain Volume

Negative thoughts and emotions are normal, and everyone has them. However, research shows that they have a significant and negative impact on *pain*. Not surprisingly, negative thoughts, such as the ones we have when we're in pain, lead to negative emotions like anger, anxiety, fear, and depression. The next step in the CBT cycle is therefore to notice how your negative thoughts make you *feel*.

When you think about your pain or illness and the way it's impacted your life, what negative emotions do you feel? (circle all that apply and add your own):

Angry	Worried	Confused
Resigned	Numb	Ashamed
Sad	Checked out	Disappointed
Grieving	Excluded	Tense
Upset	Frustrated	Furious
Worried	Depressed	Avoidant
Guilty	Self-protective	Rageful
Unsupported	Invisible	Tearful
Stressed	Annoyed	Paralyzed
Panicky	Scared	Exhausted
Unmotivated	Stuck	Hopeless
Afraid	Alone	Overwhelmed

Other words that describe how you feel:

_____

_____

_____

Emotions Live in Your Body

Emotions aren't just in your head—they also live in your body. You've likely already experienced this phenomenon many times. For example, anxiety before a deadline or a procedure might come out as stomach "butterflies," sweaty palms, stomachache, or nausea. While watching a scary movie, fear may come out as goosebumps, dry mouth, or a racing heart. Sadness and depression may make you walk and talk slowly, rob you of motivation, and make your body feel heavy and lethargic. Stress may cause hives, breakouts, headaches, or illness, and it can even make your hair turn white or fall out. Your emotions constantly and significantly impact your physical body, whether you realize it or not. This is known as the *somatic*, or bodily, aspect of emotions.

Pain Causes a Mood Crash

Chronic pain changes your life. Sometimes it *becomes* your life. Research indicates that while negative emotions amplify pain, the reverse is also true—ongoing pain can trigger a mood crash. If you've felt sad or depressed since your pain started, you're not alone: depression has been shown to co-occur with chronic pain up to 50% of the time. Not only does pain come with depression, but depression comes with pain: approximately two-thirds of people with depression report chronic pain. In addition to sadness, you may also experience grief as you mourn the loss of physical abilities, social life, sex, and mobility. This significant association between pain and depression is no coincidence. Because negative emotions trigger and exacerbate symptoms and pain, it's important to become familiar with your negative emotions and how they manifest physically. They can show up in the body in many different ways.

How do sadness and depression come out in *your* body? (circle all that apply and add your own):

Crying, tearfulness

Heaviness in body and limbs

Walking and talking slower

Sleeping more or less

Low energy

Less activity

Low motivation

Feeling like you can't get up

Loss of interest in activities

Loss of interest in sex

Anhedonia: getting less pleasure out of things than you did before

Urge to "hole up" or hide from the world

Fatigue, lethargy, physical exhaustion

Change in appetite, eating more or less

Decreased desire to go out or socialize

Staying in bed or inside

Isolating from friends and family

Irritability

Headaches, migraines

Stomachaches, nausea, vomiting

Diarrhea, constipation

Muscle aches, joint pain, unexplained body pain

Trouble concentrating

Memory difficulties

Trouble making decisions

Other ways negative emotions come out in your body:

_____

_____

_____

Coping Affects Pain

The CBT cycle then spins back around: when we think negative thoughts and feel negative feelings, we then *behave,* or act, in certain ways. These behaviors are attempts to cope, or deal with, pain and illness. A *coping behavior* can be something we do—like going to the doctor—and it can also be something we stop doing. For example, some people stop exercising because it hurts, or stop working because they feel sick and can't concentrate. Some stop seeing friends, or make a completely new group of friends with a similar illness. Some dial back on activities and spend extra time in bed or on the couch. Avoidance and withdrawal are common, and understandable, methods of coping with chronic pain.

What are some things you've started or stopped doing to cope with pain? (circle all that apply and add your own):

Visit doctors and healthcare providers

Take medicine

Spend more time in bed or on the couch

Stay in pajamas all day

Sleep during the day

Drop old hobbies, pick up new ones

Miss work

Fewer "activities of daily living" (such as cooking, driving, chores)

Fewer hobbies and pleasurable activities

Go outside less

Use screens more

Eat meals in bed

Self-soothe with food

Exercise less or not at all

Less social interaction (fewer plans, dates, parties)

Take extra medications to manage flare-ups

Guard and protect the parts that hurt by changing posture, walk, or stance

Other coping behaviors:

_____

_____

_____

Vampire Mode

What we *do* then affects how we *think* and *feel*, both emotionally and physically. Take a moment to consider what happens when you:

Stay home day after day?

Stop seeing friends?

Miss work and earn less income?

Limit favorite hobbies and enjoyable activities?

Stop exercising and moving?

Get less sunlight and fresh air?

You probably know the answer: Your mood crashes. Stress and anxiety spike as you feel more excluded, falling behind socially and professionally. As mood goes down and stress rises, the pain dial is turned up, *making pain even worse.*

This cycle is familiar to Sharon.

Sharon's Story

Sharon is a part-time teacher who struggles with chronic head and abdominal migraines. She calls her CBT pain cycle "going into Vampire Mode." Says Sharon:

"On bad pain days, I close the blinds because sunlight hurts my eyes. I call in sick to work, climb into bed, and pull the covers over my head. As the days pass, I stop seeing friends, going outside, and exercising. I dial back on hobbies like running and photography. I feel like a vampire because I come out of my room only when it's dark. After a few days, my mood crashes and I start feeling depressed. My stress and anxiety skyrocket because I'm missing work deadlines, my boss is threatening to replace me, and bills are piling up. This makes my head and stomach worse. I start thinking about how my pain is going to affect my income and livelihood, and worry that I won't qualify for disability.

"On top of that, my family and friends are moving on without me. I worry about being left out of everything and being dismissed as 'disabled.' When I think about finances, my job, my family, and my pain, the stress and anxiety get so intense that they trigger more migraines and vomiting. After a few weeks in bed, I have no motivation to leave my house.

"It feels like no one understands what I'm going through. I start thinking that if my medications haven't worked, nothing will ever work. I start believing that the rest of my life is going to be like this, that I'll be in Vampire Mode forever, that I'll lose my job, my house, and my *husband, that no one and nothing will ever help me. The more stressed and depressed I get, the worse my body feels."*

If this sounds even a little bit familiar, you're in good company—this is a common example of how thoughts, feelings, and behaviors interact when people are sick or in pain. But here's the good news: now that you're familiar with this cycle, *you have the power to break it.* That's exactly what this workbook will help you do! As you learn about your own cycle of thoughts, feelings, and coping behaviors, you'll develop new skills to control your pain dial—just as Sharon did. (She's doing wonderfully, by the way.)

Why No Pajamas?

Here's a pro tip: Even if you wake up with terrible pain and know you're not going to leave the house, *change out of pajamas anyway.* Why? Because certain behaviors, like staying in pajamas, can keep your brain stuck in "sick mode." Pain wants to consume your whole life—your job, your identity, your hobbies. The urge to stay in pajamas is your pain trying to take your power. Changing your clothes, insignificant as it seems, is a mini-revolution: one small way of taking power back. It signals to your brain that you're making a shift from disability to strength, from dysfunction to function. To be clear, this does *not* mean that on a tough day or a lazy Sunday you shouldn't lounge around in your jammies. Please do! However, changing out of pajamas—even if you hurt—is a powerful way of informing your brain that, even on days with pain, you're resilient enough to face the day.

How Stress and Anxiety Affect Pain and Health

Stress and anxiety play a significant role in pain and health, and they are *natural* and *normal* parts of the pain experience. *Stress* is typically defined as a temporary response to an external stressor that subsides once the existing threat is gone. *Anxiety* is typically defined as a sustained stress response, disproportionate to the threat of the stressor, and often focused on future events that haven't even happened yet. Anxiety can be debilitating and impair functioning across social, professional, and physical domains.

I often hear people with pain say: "Oh, but I don't have any stress or anxiety." Newsflash: pain and illness are *huge stressors* on your body. In fact, chronic pain is one of the biggest stressors there is!

Because stress and anxiety directly affect pain, it's important to be experts on these emotions. *Stress, anxiety, worry,* and *fear* are all members of the same emotion family. These emotions are your body's adaptive response to danger, helping you to survive. Back in the day, humans were hunters. While we hunted for our dinner, other animals hunted us. Your body therefore developed a system to manage emergencies: When a hungry lion approached, your body's stress-response system, including the *sympathetic nervous system* (SNS) and the *hypothalamic-pituitary-adrenal axis* (HPA)—systems that ready your body for action—released stress hormones like *adrenaline* into your bloodstream. Adrenaline sends your body into a state called *fight, flight, or freeze*. This immediately readies your body to (1) fight the lion, (2) flee from the lion and run away as fast as you can, or (3) freeze, tricking the lion into believing you're already dead. Adrenaline affects your body in many ways: it accelerates heart and respiration, halts digestion, tenses muscles, makes you feel restless, triggers feelings of fear, and produces various other sensations listed on the "Anxiety and Stress Checklist" below.

However, in today's modern world, we no longer need to hunt for our dinner with spears. Instead we buy food at the grocery store, and there aren't many lions there. But sometimes your body releases adrenaline anyway, and at inconvenient times—like when you're reading the news, faced with a deadline, or thinking about an upcoming medical procedure. *Your body also releases stress hormones when you're sick or in pain.* Pain activates your SNS stress response. Stress keeps your emergency response activated, which sensitizes your nervous system and keeps pain volume high. The more sensitive your nervous system, the louder your pain.

High stress → sensitized nervous system → higher pain volume

The more pain volume increases, the more stressed you become—and so the stress-pain cycle persists. More pain leads to more stress, more stress leads to more pain, and 'round and 'round we go.

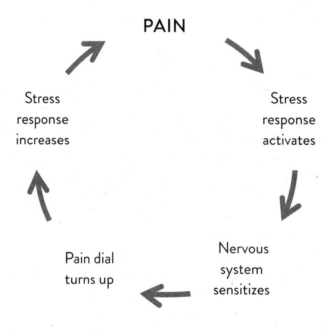

PAIN

Stress response increases

Stress response activates

Pain dial turns up

Nervous system sensitizes

Figure 3: Stress-Pain Cycle

Because your stress response gets tripped whether you're being hunted, reading about politics, or awaiting surgery, you can experience similar symptoms: hammering heart, churning stomach, rapid breathing, sweaty palms, tight back muscles, pounding head. But now you're just sitting at work, in the waiting room, or on your couch, with the urge to flee and nowhere to go. In these situations, whether you're at work or on your couch, this response is no longer adaptive or useful. Instead, it's a false alarm that causes great distress.

As if coping with pain weren't a big enough task, we also cope with various additional stressors that raise anxiety and amplify pain volume. Indeed, anxiety is on the rise worldwide. Over the last few decades, prescriptions for antianxiety drugs have more than doubled. Does everyone suddenly have a chemical imbalance or an inherited genetic anxiety disorder?

Not quite, suggests recent research. Instead, we're more likely reacting to *situational* or *environmental* triggers. That is, our anxiety may be due to stressful triggers like pandemic viruses, shelter-in-place mandates, job loss, threats of nuclear war, global terrorism, guns in schools, climate change and global warming, increasing costs of living, screens and technology, divisive politics, devastating wildfires, natural disasters…and chronic pain. Add to that the daily stressors of family conflict, grocery shopping, rush hour traffic, honking horns, crying babies, unpaid bills, insurance reimbursement, demanding bosses, a chaotic home life, arguments, and other hassles—no wonder we're so stressed! *Just like pain, anxiety and depression are also biopsychosocial*—created, amplified, and reduced by biological, psychological, social, and environmental factors.

How did reading this list of stressors make you feel?

_____

What issues trigger your anxiety and stress?

_____

_____

If you're anxious or depressed and feel like your medications aren't working, consider targeting cognitive, emotional, social, behavioral, cognitive, emotional, and situational factors like how much you exercise and play, unhealthy or abusive relationships, negative thoughts, how much you read the news and when, screen behaviors, and other biopsychosocial factors.

Anxiety and Stress Checklist

Like sadness and depression, stress and anxiety come out in the body. Because everyone is different, these emotions can manifest differently in different people. How do stress and anxiety come out in *your* body? (circle all that apply and add your own):

Feeling like you're not getting enough air

Bouncing legs, tapping feet, drumming fingers

Biting nails, picking fingers

Memory problems

Shallow or rapid breathing

Dizziness

Headaches, migraine

Tightness in chest

Desire to escape or avoid

Dry mouth

Sweating

Lightheadedness

Irritability

Fatigue, exhaustion

Stuttering

Muscle tension

Rapid heartbeat

Feeling edgy

Feeling restless

Butterflies

Trouble making decisions

Indigestion

Stomachaches

Nausea, vomiting

Fidgeting, twitching

Gas and bloating

Trouble concentrating

Blushing

Acid reflux

Mind going "blank"

Talking fast

Tight jaw, neck, shoulders

Difficulty sleeping

Rashes, hives, eczema, breakouts

Cold hands and feet

Trouble making eye contact

Muscle spasms

High energy

Difficulty finding words

Gulping, swallowing hard

Sweaty palms

Trembling, shaking

Mind racing

Bloody nose

Body or muscle pain

Crying

Irregular menstrual cycle

Hair falling out or turning gray

Unable to fall or stay asleep

Eating more or less, weight loss or gain

Grinding teeth

Diarrhea, constipation

The Relationship Between Pain, Avoidance, and More Pain

When you have chronic pain, an activated stress response might look like this:

1. **Fight**—feeling anger and rage about pain and the losses it causes; irritability; urge to hit or fight; arguments with loved ones, colleagues, or healthcare providers.

2. **Flight**—fleeing, avoiding, and escaping anything you predict or fear may cause pain. Avoiding activity, exercise, sunlight, or social events. Rejecting suggestions to move your body, especially the parts that hurt.

3. **Freeze**—the self-protective "minimal movement" response. Lying on your couch or in bed for days, weeks, or months at a time in response to pain and fear of it.

These responses are normal and understandable given the way our brains are wired to respond to stress, fear, and pain. However, when you have chronic pain, this response doesn't actually protect or help you. Instead, this cycle of fighting, fleeing, and freezing prohibits you from resuming normal functioning, prevents healthy use of muscles and tissues, and keeps pain volume turned way up. *Awareness* that your body is programmed to respond this way—and that this response isn't as helpful as it may initially seem—is the first step toward making different choices that can better help your pain.

List the ways you:

Fight

_____

_____

Flee

_____

_____

Freeze

_____

_____

Another reason to stop avoiding is that the more we avoid something that scares us—spiders, heights, physical activity—the worse anxiety gets. And the worse anxiety gets, the worse pain gets. Try this: Imagine that your anxiety is a deadly venomous snake. Every time you *avoid* the thing making you anxious, you feed that snake a big, juicy meal—making it bigger and stronger. Believe it or not, avoidance only amplifies pain and makes it harder to get back to your regularly scheduled life.

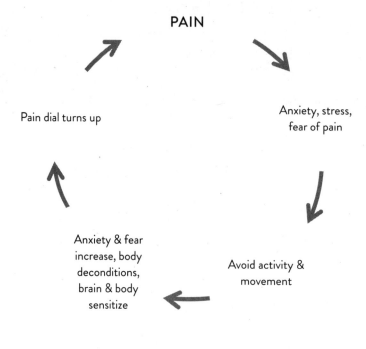

Figure 4: Avoidance-Pain Cycle

This doesn't mean you shouldn't rest or protect your body. There are absolutely times for this! But staying stuck in fear-avoidance mode long term is a surefire way to perpetuate the chronic pain cycle.

Stress and Your Immune System

This relationship between your emotional health and your physical health is so profoundly important that there's an entire branch of science devoted to it called *psychoneuroimmunology*. This is the study of how psychological processes (thoughts, emotions, behaviors), neural (brain) functioning, endocrine (hormonal) processes, and the immune system all impact and influence one another.

When you're stressed or anxious, such as when you have chronic pain or illness, your body responds in multiple ways. One is the activation of your HPA axis, triggering the release of *stress hormones* like cortisol. If you've ever doubted whether emotions directly affect health, consider this: *Cortisol suppresses your immune system.* Your immune system is your body's defense against sickness and infection, fighting off harmful pathogens like viruses and bacteria. When stress and anxiety are high, you're less able to fight off infection, more likely to get and stay sick, and more likely to experience ongoing pain.

High stress/anxiety → *high cortisol* → *weakened immune system*

In response to stress, your body also produces *pro-inflammatory cytokines*—chemicals that trigger inflammation—along with brain chemicals called *neurotransmitters* and *neuropeptides* that impact immune functioning. Together, these biological processes sensitize your pain system, amplifying warning messages from the body. If you've ever been told that stress affects pain, it's not because the pain is "all in your head"—it's because there's a real, biological link between stress, anxiety, mood, and pain.

Control Your Stress Response

When you're the boss of stress and anxiety, you're able to turn off your SNS fight-or-flight response, break the stress-pain cycle, and turn down pain volume. Skills like relaxation and mindfulness, which you'll learn in chapter 4, can help you do this. These CBT techniques activate the *parasympathetic nervous system* (PNS), your body's *rest-and-digest system.* The PNS slows your heart rate, allows your body to rest, and promotes healing. Relaxation and mindfulness techniques also reduce muscle tension, decrease cortisol and other stress hormones, and reduce blood levels of inflammatory chemicals.

Importantly, mental and physical activities that promote relaxation also tell your brain that your body is safe and doesn't require protection. Credible evidence of safety quiets that ringing false alarm and lowers pain volume.

Stress/danger → *SNS on, PNS off* → *pain volume high*

Relaxation/safety → *SNS off, PNS on* → *pain volume lower*

Trauma and Pain

There's a well-established and strong association between trauma and chronic pain. Research suggests that repeated exposure to trauma, especially in childhood—including maltreatment, abuse, assault, neglect, exposure to domestic violence and crime, parental mental illness or parental loss, and other early traumas—can leave an "imprint" on the brain that increases vulnerability to chronic pain. Indeed, studies on adverse childhood experiences (ACEs) reveal that experiencing traumatic events in childhood is a major risk factor for developing chronic pain and illness in adulthood. ACEs are also associated with anxiety and depression in adulthood, which, in turn, are associated with pain and health problems.

Trauma during adulthood is also a risk factor for developing chronic pain. This includes the trauma of emotional and physical abuse, domestic violence, death of a loved one, combat and war, a miscarriage, a car accident, or *medical trauma*—the trauma that can arise as a result of medical issues, treatments, or procedures gone awry. It can even stem from the first time you were held down as a child to get an injection. Chronic pain in adulthood can also be triggered by the memory or reactivation of a childhood trauma. This is why pain sometimes feels worse when people return to the place of their initial injury or trauma, or any place that reminds them of it. While not everyone who's lived through a trauma has post-traumatic stress disorder (PTSD), it's worth noting that the "S" in PTSD stands for "stress"—a major contributor to chronic pain.

The link between trauma and pain is not a coincidence: it's biology. Traumatic experiences put the brain on high alert, training it to chronically scan the environment for potential dangers so that it can better protect you. The human body also responds to trauma with a heightened, intensified stress response, even after the stressor is gone. The nervous system, stuck in survival mode, continues to produce stress hormones like cortisol, which suppress the immune system and limit the body's ability to heal. This can lead to chronic physical symptoms like pain and fatigue. An activated stress response plus a brain on high alert for danger are a recipe for high pain volume. Since emotions live in your body, and since chronic pain is often a sign of unresolved trauma, treating trauma is often an important part of chronic-pain work.

While treating trauma is beyond the scope of this workbook, let's check in:

Have you experienced trauma in your lifetime?   (circle) Y / N

How do you feel physically and emotionally when you think about the trauma(s) you've endured?

_____

_____

Do you suspect that unresolved trauma may play a role in your pain?   (circle) Y / N

What was happening in your life at the time of pain onset?

_____

_____

_____

Was anything about these circumstances traumatizing or associated with a traumatic memory?

_____

_____

Because the link between trauma and chronic pain is so strong, it's highly recommended that you find a therapist you like and trust to help you heal. Having a trained professional to guide and support you is critical, especially if you've never processed trauma before. Trauma-focused CBT, prolonged exposure therapy, cognitive processing therapy, and eye-movement desensitization reprocessing (EMDR) are a few established interventions. Consider joining a support group and check out the trauma books in the "Resources" section near the end of this book. Since your emotional health is inextricably connected to your physical health, start healing from the inside out.

Anger and Pain

Chronic pain is associated with significant loss—loss of function, loss of activity, loss of routines, loss of relationships, and loss of control over one's body. This normally and naturally generates feelings of sadness, mourning, resentment, and _anger_. Anger is also a standard reaction to trauma.

If you experience anger, this emotion is a valid response to pain and loss. Anger can be an unpleasant experience, however, and can lead to additional negative emotions like guilt and shame. Your anger may have multiple targets: your insurance company, failed treatments, healthcare providers, the boss who won't provide accommodations, or unsupportive family members. It may be hard to know where to direct your anger or who to blame, so the anger may sometimes explode everywhere—on random drivers on the road, on someone walking too slowly on the sidewalk, or on that door that just won't open. Conversely, your anger may turn inward. Inward-facing anger can manifest as self-loathing, rage toward a painful body part, self-mutilation, substance use, and other self-harming behaviors. These behaviors are often attempts to cope with, and distract from, anger.

There are healthy and less healthy ways to deal with anger. What are some of your less healthy coping mechanisms?

_____

_____

There are also healthier ways of dealing with anger. These might include redirecting that energy elsewhere—like ripping a phone book—or getting the anger out by exercising, lifting weights, writing, drawing, or talking to someone.

Think of two healthy ways you can manage your anger:

1. _____

2. _____

It's possible to heal from and to manage anger. As distressing as it may be, anger isn't permanent and it doesn't define you. "Angry" isn't who you *are*—it's just how you *feel*. At its core, anger is a just a transient emotion—a harmless collection of brain chemicals and physical sensations—and it has no more power than any other emotion. Anger offers up important information for us to notice and use for healing: you're hurting and need soothing.

Like every other emotion, anger lives not just in your head, but also in your body. For example, your face might get red-hot, your hands curl into fists, your jaw tighten, your muscles tense as if ready to spring, your head pound, and your temples throb.

Where do you typically feel anger in your body?

_____

_____

Anger is a normal, human emotion. You can't ignore it (at least, not if you want to be healthy!) and you can't destroy it. The best you can do is acknowledge and cope with it. The shame and guilt you feel aren't helping, either—if anything, they only make you feel worse, perpetuating a self-hating, angry cycle. One strategy you can use is to start treating your anger with kindness and compassion instead of hate and loathing.

HEALING ANGER

If you loathe and feel ashamed of your anger, try using imagery to change your relationship with it, transforming it from a dangerous, hateful monster to a gentle, helpless animal, a creature you can love and manage. For example, practice imagining that your anger is a furry dog with big, sweet eyes. (Sound silly? Try it anyway!) Whenever you hear your anger yowling, instead of raging at it, hating it, and stuffing it into a tiny cage, put him on a leash and take him outside for a walk. Speak to him soothingly and kindly in a voice you'd use with someone you love. Take him for long runs, letting all the hot, angry steam seep out of your body. Give him a warm, soothing bath or a cold, bracing shower. Put him under a warm blanket and let him watch movies. Sit down and write about your anger, or call a friend and vent, and let him sit on your lap. Rip phone books into tiny shreds while he watches, delightedly wagging his tail. It's healthy and important to "externalize" your anger—to recognize that this emotion lives in you but is not you, and that it needs your help, kindness, and attention in order to be soothed.

Picture your anger as an innocent, sweet animal. What does it look like?

_____

Name three ways you can kindly, compassionately take care of your anger. What are some strategies you can use to help him when he needs you most?

1. _____

2. _____

3. _____

If your experience with anger is hurting you or the people you love, there's no time to waste. Try these strategies this week and practice them daily. Find a therapist trained in anger management, trauma, PTSD, or "nonviolent communication" to help you navigate your anger. Join a gym and try kick-boxing, stockpile phone books for ripping, and make plans to take your anger for lots of walks. Check the "Resources" section near the end of this book for additional books and resources.

What Good Are Emotions?

Some people try to push negative emotions away, ignore them, reject them, or squash them. Research shows that suppressing and masking emotions can actually lead to more pain and physical symptoms. It's therefore important to understand the role that emotions serve and how they help and protect us.

Why do we even have emotions?

1. EMOTIONS GIVE US INFORMATION ABOUT OURSELVES.

- Like pain, emotions are adaptive. They help us survive by providing useful information about ourselves and the world around us.

- Emotions help us "act on instinct" rather than overthinking. This can save time in dangerous situations. If a car is approaching and your life is in danger, that fear you instantly feel saves your life by urging you to move!

- The ability to recognize an emotion helps you get your needs met. If you're scared, you can find ways to feel safe. If you know you're sad, you can do something to feel better. If you don't understand your emotions, you won't know how to cope with them.

Example: Cal got into a taxi and noticed that the car reeked of alcohol. The driver was weaving as he drove and crossed over to the wrong side of the road. Cal's palms got sweaty, his heart started racing, his stomach lurched, and his chest felt tight. He recognized that he felt afraid because he was in danger. He asked the driver to stop the car, got out, called a friend to pick him up—and instantly felt better.

Name a time you were able to take care of yourself because you were aware of how you felt:

_____

_____

2. EMOTIONS GIVE US INFORMATION ABOUT OTHERS.

- Emotions are communicated by facial expressions, body language, words, and sounds. Correctly interpreting this information gives us the ability to better understand and communicate with those around us.

- Emotions tell us who's safe and who's threatening—who to approach and who to avoid.

- Emotions tell us what other people need. If your child is crying, you can comfort her. If your friend is yelling, you can give him space to calm down.

Example: Ryan saw a man on the sidewalk throwing glass bottles and shouting, realized the man was angry and aggressive, and crossed to the other side of the street to stay safe.

When has an emotion protected you?

_____

When did you know someone was angry just by reading his or her body language? How did this affect what you said or did?

_____

_____

3. EMOTIONS GIVE OTHERS INFORMATION ABOUT US.

- The way you express and communicate your emotions influences the way others react to you, and helps others respond appropriately. If you're crying, you might need a hug; if you're anxious, you might need reassurance.

- People tend to "lean in" when you're sad, laugh with you when you're happy, and back off when you're angry and need space. Expressing how you feel helps you get your needs met.

Example: Gabriella had had a hard day. She was stressed and frustrated. Her husband kept nagging her to help with dinner and she felt like she was going to explode. She finally turned to him and said, "I'll help you with that in a few minutes. Right now, I'm feeling overwhelmed and just need to be alone." Her husband backed off and gave her some space.

What strategies effectively help you get your needs met when you're upset, anxious, overwhelmed, or in pain?

_____

_____

4. EMOTIONS VALIDATE AND REWARD US.

- When emotions motivate you to engaging in healthy behaviors that help you to function and thrive, this helps you trust your own instincts.

- Positive emotions increase levels of brain chemicals that further improve your mood and make you feel good. When you laugh, you actually feel happier!

- Positive emotions feel so good that they encourage us to repeat certain behaviors.

Example: Going for a bike ride with friends made Audrey feel so energized, strong, and happy that she wanted to go again the next day!

Name one positive behavior that feels rewarding:

_____

Rather than hating emotions, feeling ashamed of them, or pushing them away, try to listen to them. It's their job to give you information and help you, not hurt you. This book is full of healthy ways to work with difficult emotions.

Pain Triggers

Once you understand the relationship between thoughts, feelings, coping behaviors, and pain, the next step is to break the cycle. One way to transform the CBT pain cycle is to identify the things that trigger—or set off—your pain. A *trigger* is a difficult situation, emotion, or event that causes pain to increase. Triggers, like everything else relating to pain, are biopsychosocial.

Pain triggers can be biological (a sprain, constipation, an infection); social (family conflict, job loss, environmental stressors); and psychological (rooted in negative thoughts [also known as *cognitions*], memories, emotions, and behaviors).

Adam's, Gina's, and Paul's Stories

Adam was recovering from back surgery. He got into an argument with his wife about making the kids' dinner (social trigger) and became angry and frustrated (emotional trigger). He felt the anger in his body, his muscles got hot and tight (biological trigger), and his back started spasming.

Gina is another example of how different types of triggers can work together to cause a pain flare. She believed that nothing could cure her fibromyalgia (cognitive trigger), which made her feel depressed and hopeless (emotional trigger). She stayed home for weeks without work, friends, or distractions (behavioral trigger) and started feeling significantly worse.

Paul's initial trigger was biological—he was constipated and hadn't had a bowel movement in three days (biological trigger), which caused intense abdominal pain, bloating, and discomfort. This led him to strain every time he went to the bathroom (behavioral trigger), triggering a flare-up of hemorrhoids and anorectal pain. The ongoing constipation also spiked anxiety and frustration (emotional trigger), which further turned up the pain dial.

What *emotions* trigger your pain? (circle all that apply and add your own)

Frustration

Anger

Stress

Anxiety

Loneliness

Sadness

_____

_____

What *social* or *environmental situations* trigger your pain?

Arguing with family members

Threat of job loss

Unsupportive friends

Missing out on activities because you're sick

Watching the news

Inadequate access to healthcare

_____

_____

What *biological factors* trigger your pain?

Not getting enough sleep

Poor diet

Dehydration

Bright lights and loud noises

Poor circulation

Lifting heavy objects

Lack of exercise and muscle atrophy

_____

_____

Know Your Pain Recipe

In order to cook a delicious meal, you must follow a particular recipe—ingredients, oven temperature, cooking time—to get your dish just right. For example, if you want to bake brownies, skipping steps or ignoring baking instructions will give you burned, dry, inedible brownies, and nobody wants one of those.

Pain works similarly. Just as there's a recipe for brownies, there's also a recipe for pain. Your *high-pain recipe* is a list of all the ingredients, or triggers, that go into creating a high-pain day. These can be anything off the biopsychosocial menu: stressors, current events, situations at work or home, thoughts, memories, emotions, poor sleep, inadequate nutrition, or toxic company. Everyone's pain recipe is different, but when combined, these ingredients combust to trigger, maintain, and exacerbate pain.

Just as you have a high-pain recipe, you also have a *low-pain recipe*. A low-pain recipe is all the biopsychosocial ingredients that go into creating a low-pain day. How can you exert some control over which kind of day you're going to have? One technique is to closely examine your low- and high-pain days and notice the ingredients for each.

For example, Emma noticed that certain situations, thoughts, feelings, and events contributed to feeling awful, while others contributed to feeling a bit better. She tracked her triggers and noticed the following high-pain ingredients:

Emma's High-Pain Recipe

- Skipping meals, poor nutrition

- Being "out of balance": hungry, overworked, insufficient sleep

- Overcommitting: too many activities, responsibilities, deadlines, and tasks

- High stress

- Anxiety and frustration about pain

- Not having time to relax, exercise, or have fun

Emma's Low-Pain Recipe

- Three meals a day plus snacks (being well-fed, eating a nutritious diet)

- Being balanced: sleeping well, eating regularly, maintaining a balanced workload

- Saying "no": limiting extra work, responsibilities, and activities at home

- Low stress

- Using coping strategies to manage anxiety and frustration about pain

- Scheduling time to engage in self-care: exercise, relax, knit, embroider, create art, journal

Ideas for Ingredient Changes

Emma noticed that her overly hectic lifestyle frequently resulted in a recipe for high pain. One thing that helped immensely was replacing some high-pain ingredients with low-pain ingredients. These were her ideas:

- Schedule one hour of protected "relaxation time" after work, plus two hours on weekends to walk and draw.

- Set an alarm at mealtimes to prevent skipping meals, and keep snacks in work bag.

- Go to bed earlier, sleep later on weekends.

- Say "no" to extra responsibilities at work and at home.

- Hire a babysitter one evening a week and go out with girlfriends.

Enter your high-pain and low-pain recipes (bonus brownie recipe!):

Your Pain Recipe

Brownie Recipe	High-Pain Recipe	Low-Pain Recipe
1½ cups flour		
2 cups sugar		
4 eggs		
¾ teaspoon baking soda		

½ teaspoon salt		
1 cup butter		
½ cup cocoa powder		

List five ideas for replacing high-pain ingredients with low-pain ingredients:

1. _____

2. _____

3. _____

4. _____

5. _____

Release Negative Emotions: How to Teakettle

Negative emotions live in the body, but we don't want them to stay there. It's therefore important to learn how to release them. Because pain is both physical and emotional, addressing and releasing negative emotions can help you effectively manage pain. One way to do this is to *teakettle*. What is teakettling, you ask? First, answer this:

Q: What would happen to a teakettle if it didn't have a hole for the steam to escape?

A: The steam would have nowhere to go. The pressure inside the teakettle would rise, and rise, and rise, until—BOOM!—it exploded.

Similarly, negative emotions need a place to go. If you don't find healthy outlets to release them, they find ways to come out on their own. Negative emotions can come out in your body as muscle tension, back pain, stomachaches, vomiting, rashes, or chronic pain. A great way to remedy this is to "teakettle": let out, or express, your emotions in a healthy way. (That's why it's called "venting"!) This way, pent-up emotions won't come out as physical symptoms or pain. Better yet, they won't get stuck inside of you to begin with.

Here are some great ways to teakettle:

- Talk to someone. Put feelings into words and release them.

- Write or journal. Writing takes emotions out of your head and body, translates them into words, and releases them on paper.

- Create art. Drawing, painting, and other arts transform emotions into colors, shapes, and images.

- Dance. Dancing and moving help channel emotions into creative physical expression.

- Perform. Theater, singing, and acting are outlets for expressing and releasing emotion.

- Play an instrument. Transform your emotions into music.

- Exercise. Moving and sweating release emotional energy.

- Other ideas: Let yourself cry. Scream in your car. Rip a phone book to shreds. Punch a pillow.

Your ideas for teakettling:

_____

_____

_____

_____

One way you'll teakettle today:

_____

Write Your Pain Story

Expressive writing—writing about the emotional impact of pain and difficult life events—is a great way to teakettle. Research shows that this type of writing can actually boost immune functioning and even change pain. Writing can help you express and release strong emotions, process difficult events, and organize your thoughts, all of which can help you heal.

For this activity, you'll have the opportunity to write your pain story. Your pain story includes the history of your pain and how you feel about every part of your journey. You can write for a few minutes or a few hours. As you tell your story, consider the following questions: How and when did your pain begin? What was going on in your life at the time? How have pain and illness impacted your ability to work, play, and function? What treatments have you tried, and how many doctors have you seen? What have the costs been, financially and emotionally? Most importantly: write about how all of this makes you *feel.* Use emotion words, as many as you've got.

Your pain story:

_____

_____

_____

_____

_____

_____

_____

_____

_____

_____

_____

_____

_____

_____

_____

_____

_____

_____

_____

Use additional pages as necessary or get a journal. Consider making expressive writing a part of your daily life.

Conclusion

CBT is an evidence-based treatment for chronic pain that targets triggers, thoughts, emotions, and coping behaviors. The limbic system, your brain's emotion center, plays a critical role in the experience of pain. Emotions don't just live in your head, they also come out in your body, directly impacting health and pain. Negative emotions like stress, anxiety, depression, and anger change hormones, neurotransmitters, and brain pathways to amplify pain, as does trauma. Effective CBT-based methods for managing pain include identifying biopsychosocial triggers, learning your personal pain recipe, releasing negative emotions by "teakettling," and targeting unhealthy coping behaviors such as avoidance and withdrawal. Just as we can change pain by changing triggers and emotions, we can also change pain using behavioral techniques. The next chapter on "pain-control strategies" will show you how!

CHAPTER 3

Pain-Control Strategies

It's understandable to believe that pain needs to resolve *before* you can resume activities: pain reduction first, activity second. Indeed, this is the appropriate response to acute pain. If you have an acute injury or illness—a broken leg, a severe fever—your adaptive, accurate instinct is to stop, rest, and heal.

However, the effective approach to chronic pain is totally counterintuitive. To effectively treat chronic pain, the process is the opposite: first you gradually, slowly resume activity and function, exposing the brain and body to low levels of stimulation, and *then* desensitization occurs.

Act First, Feel Changes Later: How to Work Backward

To retrain a sensitized brain, it's critically important to fight the instinct to stop all activity and movement. Avoidance, withdrawal, and long periods of rest only contribute to the cycle of stiffness, muscle atrophy, subsequent anxiety and depression, and more pain. To start feeling better, try to *work backward* and resume activities first. Once you start moving, getting more sunlight, seeing friends, and reengaging in hobbies and pleasurable activities, the more likely your mood is to go up, stress and anxiety to go down, and pain volume to gradually decrease. If this sounds scary or uncomfortable, that's a normal reaction—in fact, it's biological. That's your highly sensitive pain alarm falsely warning you that something dangerous and harmful will happen if you move. Treating chronic pain requires constantly pushing the "off" button on this alarm, reminding your brain that your body is safe—despite the very real pain you feel.

Here's how working backward worked for Jack:

Jack's Story

Jack is a biologist and former soccer player who struggles with crippling rheumatoid arthritis. It caused terrible joint pain that required surgery. He'd stopped commuting into the city for work, and had also stopped playing soccer with his pickup team, which was his stress release and a source of great joy. He figured he'd have to wait for the pain to go away—presumably, after surgery—before he could go back. But once he learned the strategy of working backward, he decided he'd waited long enough. He missed enjoying his life.

Jack decided to start physical therapy along with CBT to regain strength, muscle tone, and body confidence. After a few months, he went back to the soccer field and just walked around the perimeter, gently kicking a ball. His buddies were glad to see him. After a few weeks of walking and training, his physical therapist gave him the green light to jog the perimeter of the field. He stayed to watch the game and afterwards joined his team for dinner. It felt like medicine, and resuming activity actually lessened his pain. The more he did, the more he felt like he could do.

Overcoming Inertia

The concept of *inertia* comes from a law of physics that states that "objects in motion tend to stay in motion," while "objects at rest tend to stay at rest." This law applies to humans, too. It can be hard to overcome the pull of inertia, change behaviors, and start doing something new—even harder when you're in pain. But have you ever noticed that once you're off the couch and moving, the energy required to keep going is much less than was required to get up? Conversely, the longer you stay on that couch, the stronger the pull is to keep lying there. The steps in this book are designed to help you overcome inertia and successfully start working backward!

MOTIVATION ASSESSMENT

Before we dive into pain-control strategies, it's helpful to honor hesitations and fears. It's normal to feel ambivalent about starting a new pain program. Assessing the pros and cons can affect engagement and motivation, and even influence outcomes.

Is your current pain-management plan working? Why or why not?

_____

_____

_____

What has pain taken from you that you want to take back?

1. _____

2. _____

3. _____

Name one way this book might help you.

_____

The "Decisional Balance" exercise below will help you determine the benefits ("pros") and costs ("cons") of behavior change. Read the statement on the left, then consider possible advantages and disadvantages. Here's Samuel's decisional balance:

Samuel's Decisional Balance

	Disadvantages (cons)	Advantages (pros)
No change: Keep my old pain-management program.	If I keep doing what I've been doing, my pain will stay the same. What I'm doing isn't working or I'd be better by now.	My old way of managing pain is familiar. I know what to expect. I don't have to change my routine.
Make a change: Adopt a new pain program and actively use this workbook.	Change is scary and unfamiliar. I don't need therapy. What if my pain gets worse?	This new program could improve my pain and my life. It could enable me to play with my grandkids again. I have nothing to lose.

Your Decisional Balance

	Disadvantages (cons)	Advantages (pros)
No change: Keep my old pain-management program.		
Make a change: Adopt a new pain program and actively use this workbook.		

Circle the bottom right square (advantages of change) and the top left square (disadvantages of no change). These statements embody the mind frame that's most likely to motivate you to transform your pain and reclaim your life! Recite these statements to yourself any time you encounter physical or emotional obstacles, notice that you're resistant, or feel stuck.

Goal-Setting

Engaging in activities by working backward can help you break the cycle of pain and illness. So how do you decide where to start? The first step is to *establish a goal*. Committing to a goal can motivate and ready you to take the necessary steps to change your pain.

No matter what your goals are—be they physical, social, or work-related—make them more achievable by following these steps. First, state your goals in terms of what you *do* want instead of what you *don't* want. For example, "I don't want to be trapped at home" keeps your brain stuck in the negative and lacks a plan for forward motion. Instead, try starting with: "Go outside more." Then, follow these goal-setting steps:

- **Be realistic.** Make your goals meaningful, realistic, and achievable. Setting unrealistic goals only results in frustration. For example, instead of "Feel better by June," try "Use three CBT strategies today."

- **Be specific.** State your goal using units of *measurement*—time of day, quantity, and duration. For example, instead of "Be more social," which is broad and vague, try "Call one friend on Tuesday at noon." Instead of "Go back to work," try "Go to work for one hour three days this week."

- **Break your big goal into smaller steps.** It's okay to dream big! Identify your overarching dream goals and pursue them. Just make sure to break down these big goals into smaller steps. This makes them less intimidating and more achievable. Small steps are also more trackable, so you can see where you've been and where you're going. For example, if your goal is to resume mountain biking, your small steps might look like this: "Week 1—bike 10 mins daily at 1 pm. Week 2—bike 15 mins daily at 1 pm. Week 3—bike 20 mins daily at 1 pm."

- **Pick a practical starting point.** Identify a realistic starting point that doesn't sound overwhelming. Starting small gives your plastic brain and body a chance to gradually adjust to change. For example, if your goal is to resume running, don't start by running five miles after a month of not moving. Your body won't be used to it, and overexertion can trigger pain. Instead, set a small, measurable starting goal, like "Walk 15 mins every day for one week."

- **Measure progress.** Keep a chart to track daily progress. It's rewarding and encouraging to watch your improvement. Celebrate every small victory, and feel proud of every accomplishment!

- **Anticipate obstacles.** Anticipate obstacles before they happen, and troubleshoot solutions in advance. This way, you're ahead of the game. Ask yourself, *What might get in the way of achieving this goal?* These could be thoughts, fears, physical challenges, or practical obstacles like not having a car.

- **Earn rewards!** Rewards help motivate us and move us forward. For example, some people work hard to earn money, while others work hard for recognition and accolades. Some people will work for chocolate! Rewards are different for different people. Set up a system to reward yourself for accomplishing each small goal. Rewards can be attending a concert, money toward a guitar, a shopping spree, or a vacation.

Add your goals in the space below. Use Lily's examples to guide you.

Lily's big dream goal: Resume Irish dancing

Your big dream goal: _____

Lily's first small step (goal 1): 1. Attend one dance rehearsal this week and just watch.

Your first small step (goal 1): 1. _____

When Lily will take that first step: After work today at 6 pm.

When you'll take that first step: _____

Lily's next three realistic, specific steps (goals 2–4):

2. Email dance teacher today at noon.

3. Attend weekly dance rehearsals Fridays at 6 pm.

4. Practice dancing at home for 10 minutes 3 days this week.

Your next three realistic, specific steps (include date, time, and units of measurement):

2. _____

3. _____

4. _____

Lily's Progress Chart (X = complete)

	Mon.	Tues.	Wed.	Thurs.	Fri.	Sat.	Sun.
Dream goal: Resume Irish dancing							
Goal 1: Attend rehearsal, just watch	X						
Goal 2: Email teacher	X						
Goal 3: Weekly rehearsal					X		
Goal 4: Dance 3 days for 10 mins		X	X			X	

Your Progress Chart

	Mon.	Tues.	Wed.	Thurs.	Fri.	Sat.	Sun.
Dream goal:							
Goal 1:							
Goal 2:							
Goal 3:							
Goal 4:							

You can download a copy of this chart at http://www.newharbinger.com/46448.

Lily's potential obstacles and solutions:

Obstacle 1: The dance teacher might not email me back.

Solution 1: If she doesn't, I'll go to her studio.

Obstacle 2: I'll likely get tired and have pain.

Solution 2: I'll take frequent breaks and bring an ice pack.

Your potential obstacles and solutions:

Obstacle 1: _____

Solution 1: _____

Obstacle 2: _____

Solution 2: _____

Obstacle 3: _____

Solution 3: _____

Lily's reward ideas: If I complete all of this week's goals, I'll earn a new recipe book and mixing bowl.

Your reward ideas: _____

_____

Goals for Healing

In addition to establishing physical, social, and career goals, take a moment to establish goals for healing. Healing goals are different for everyone. For example, your goal may be to get healthy enough to leave the hospital. It may be to reduce pain enough to drive. Or your healing goal may be to eliminate a particular symptom. "Healthy" and "healed" mean different things to different people.

What does "healthy" mean to you?

_____

_____

What's your primary goal for healing? (*reduce pain, manage symptoms, resume a particular function or activity*)

_____

_____

What does "able to function" mean to you? (*able to walk with crutches, able to resume karate, able to spend time with friends*)

_____

_____

Consider your goals at different pain levels. What activities do you aspire to accomplish if your pain is:

0/10? (On a scale of 0–10, 0 = no pain, 5 = moderate pain, 10 = extreme pain.)

_____

_____

2/10?

_____

_____

4/10?

_____

_____

6/10?

_____

_____

8/10?

_____

_____

10/10?

_____

_____

Once you've established your goals, you're ready to take the next step in pain mastery! Pacing is a great place to begin.

Pacing: How to Resume Work and Play

An important strategy for desensitizing your sensitive nervous system and resuming functioning is called *pacing*. Pacing is a graded exposure activity that can help you reduce pain flares, do more of what's important to you, conserve energy for activities you value, and feel more in control of your life. You can use this skill to resume hobbies, exercise, activities of daily living, or to return to work.

On days with pain, some people protect themselves by resting, reducing activity, and staying home. This can last for weeks, months, or even years. Many even develop a fear of movement called *kinesiophobia* (from *kinesia* or *kinesis*, meaning "movement," and *phobia*, which means "fear of"). While avoiding and withdrawing from movement and activity seem reasonable and understandable, resting for too long actually makes it *harder* to return to the activities you love. Your body gets stiffer and less fit, muscle tension and soreness increase, motivation decreases, your nervous system stays hypersensitive, and movement and activity become even more painful. On top of that, avoiding physical and social activity actually *increases* anxiety and pain-related fear, which then turn up the pain dial. The cycle of inactivity as a result of pain looks like this:

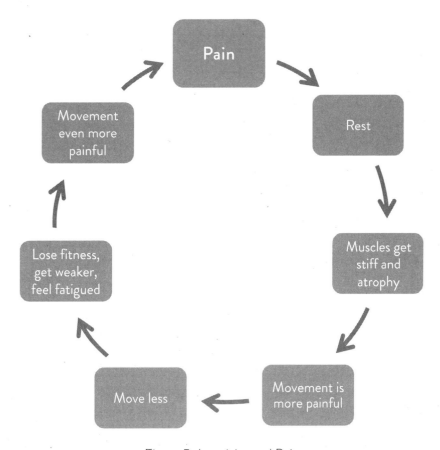

Figure 5: Inactivity and Pain

On low-pain days, some people do the opposite. They're so excited to have less pain that they try to do as much as possible. They go shopping, catch up on work and chores, go for a run, then spend the rest of the day with family and friends. But what happens when you push yourself too hard?

Ugh. Pain! You may crash and not be able to get out of bed for days. This cycle of intense over-activity and underactivity *decreases* your overall functionality. This is the dotted line you see in the diagram below (Figure 6). This boom-and-bust, up-and-down cycle actually results in less activity over time rather than more, because it wears out both your body and your resolve.

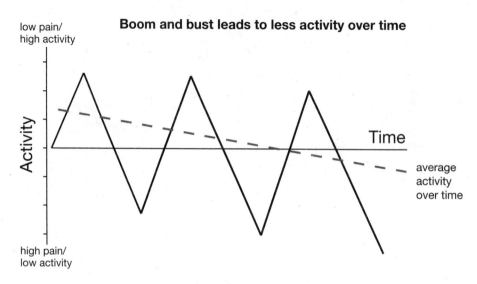

Figure 6: Boom and Bust

One way to find a balance between doing too little and too much is to try *pacing*. When you pace yourself, you engage in a regular, daily level of activity somewhere between doing nothing (too little) and doing everything (way too much). Exposing your brain and body to carefully calibrated amounts of stimulation and movement over time can result in a gradual increase in activity and functioning.

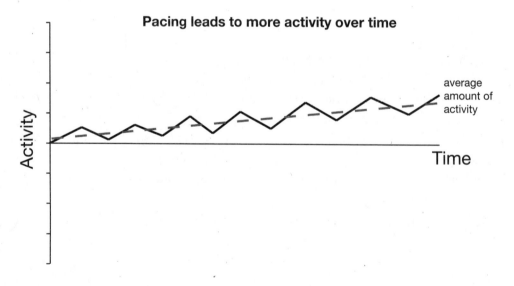

Figure 7: Pacing Improvement

Pacing is like warming up an old car after it's been sitting outside in the winter snow for too long. The engine has become cold and clunky from disuse and needs to warm up before it can perform well. Your sluggish car can't drive cross-country the instant you turn it on! First it needs to warm up in the driveway, and then do some practice laps around the block. Once the engine is warm and used to moving, it can go longer distances. This is true for you, too. Think of pacing as a way to gradually warm up your brain and body.

Pacing = Brain- and Body-Warming

Even if you've been inactive for months, you can warm your brain and body starting today. *Now.* Pick any activity! You can pace to resume activities of daily living, like grocery shopping or mowing. You can pace to exercise or restart your favorite hobby, like Irish dance, soccer, or even sewing.

Note that pacing is *not* the same as "pushing through the pain" or the concept of "no pain, no gain." Rather, pacing is a method of graded activity and exposure that requires finding a safe, comfortable starting point—even if it's just two minutes of activity—then stopping at the designated stopping point. It also incorporates taking breaks to stretch and rest.

Pacing Brainstorm

What *physical activities* are you willing to try this week? It can be something you need to do, like cleaning the house, or something you *want* to do, like ice skating or making fudge. Try to pick a valued or prioritized activity that feels like a good place to start.

Walk outside	Trip to the post office	Fix things around the house
Cook dinner	Vacuum	
Yoga	Go out with friends	Jumping jacks
Hike	Walk the dog around the block	Take family out for a nice meal
Dance class	Take the car to the shop	Online exercise class
Laundry	Swim	Water aerobics at the YMCA
Lift light weights	Ride a bike	Drive to the beach
Soccer	Garden	Grocery shopping
Walk to the mailbox		

Your ideas for pacing:

1. _____

2. _____

3. _____

4. _____

Activity Pacing

The trick to pacing is to set realistic, measurable goals that are meaningful to you, and then slowly work your way up to them—bit by bit. First, pick an activity you'd like to try but have been unable to do because of pain or illness. Then create a *pacing plan*.

Here's my example:

Step 1. Set a goal. Pick a physical activity you'd like to resume or try.

Hike in the redwoods

Step 2. State your ultimate dream goal for this activity using specific measurements like time, duration, and frequency.

Hike outdoors for one hour, 3 days a week.

Step 3. Measure the length of time you can do this activity comfortably on a low-pain day, and then on a high-pain day.

On a low-pain day, I can hike for 20 minutes. On a high-pain day, I can hike for only 4 minutes.

Step 4. Calculate the average by adding these together, then dividing the total by two.

20 (low pain) + 4 (high pain) = 24 minutes (total)

24 (total) ÷ 2 = 12 minutes (average)

Step 5. Once you have an average amount of time you can do this activity, subtract a few minutes to give yourself a cushion. This will be your *baseline,* or the amount of time you will do this activity every day—whether it's a high-pain day or a low-pain day.

$$Baseline = Daily\ activity\ goal$$

Don't do more, and try not to do too much less. This will prevent you from becoming inactive and also from overexerting yourself. Most importantly, it will help your plastic brain desensitize.

12 minutes (average) 2-minutes (cushion) = 10 minutes (daily baseline)

Step 6. Plan to take "rest and stretch" breaks after a set number of minutes, and establish the length of your break. You can take multiple breaks as needed. The length of your break should shorten over time as your strength and stamina increase.

Break schedule: one 2-minute break every 5 minutes.

Step 7. Each week, add a few minutes to your activity, depending on your tolerance, until you reach your ultimate goal. This is your weekly *activity increase.* Some people may be able to add ten minutes while some will add two. Don't judge yourself for starting slowly—creating an individualized, graded exposure plan that feels good to you is very important.

I'll increase hiking by 2 minutes weekly until I reach my goal. Since my baseline is 10 minutes, I'll hike in the redwoods for 12 minutes next week, and the following week I'll aim to hike for 14 minutes.

Over time your brain will respond a little less to those loud, false-alarm warning messages you've been getting all the time, because you're slowly warming it up like an engine. It will unlearn the emergency response to harmless stimuli, like gardening or hiking, that make you *hurt* but don't cause *harm.* Your body will get used to moving, your muscles will get stronger, and fitness will increase. You'll get better at tolerating whatever activities you choose, even on days when you feel sick or have some pain.

For example, I'll hike outdoors for ten minutes every day during week one, even if I have some pain. There will be times I want to hike more (on days I feel awesome), and times I want to stay in bed and not hike at all (on days I feel awful). But I'll use my pacing plan to accomplish ten minutes of activity every day, which will help my brain rewire and enable my body to get healthy and strong again.

Schedule Breaks

Taking *breaks* is an important part of pacing. Build a "rest and stretch" break into your pacing schedule, making sure to pause before pain gets too intense. Drink water, take deep breaths, listen to music, pet the cat, stretch. Change your position and posture to increase tolerance to movement. It's also useful to get support by asking someone to pace with you. For example, if I'm having a tough day, I'll ask a friend to hike with me for company and cheer me on. Having loved ones pace with you can make it more tolerable and enjoyable.

Create your own pacing plan for this week. For subsequent weeks, copy a blank handout from this book and fill in new pacing goals as they change (and they will!). Download a blank copy of this activity pacing plan at http://www.newharbinger.com/46448.

Your Activity Pacing Plan

Step 1. Set a goal. Pick a physical activity you'd like to resume or try. You can make it aspirational or practical, as long as it's personally meaningful.

_____

Step 2. State your ultimate dream goal for this activity, using specific measurements like time, duration, and frequency.

_____

_____

Step 3. Measure the length of time (in minutes) you can do this activity comfortably on a low-pain day, then on a high-pain day.

Low-pain day: _____

High-pain day: _____

Step 4. Calculate the average by adding these times together, and then divide the total by two.

Low pain _____ + high pain _____ = _____ (total)

Total _____ ÷ 2 = _____ (average)

Step 5. Once you have an average amount of time you can do that activity, subtract a few minutes to give yourself a cushion. This will be your daily baseline.

Average _____ – _____ minutes (cushion) = _____ (daily baseline)

Step 6. Plan to take a "rest and stretch" break after a set number of minutes, and establish the length of your break. This number will change from week to week as your strength and stamina increase.

Scheduled break every _____ number of minutes.

Each break will be _____ minutes.

Step 7. Determine your weekly activity increase. Aim to add a few (approximately 2–5) minutes to your activity each week, depending on your tolerance, until you reach your ultimate goal.

Your weekly activity increase: _____ minutes

The Importance of Walking

One of the most important activities you can resume is *walking*. Walking lubricates your joints for easier motion, gets blood flowing, desensitizes the brain and body to low-impact movement, and can increase strength and mobility. It can also increase your functioning. Walking is so important that many pain programs recommend targeting it as the first pacing goal. Therefore, try to set aside time to walk every day. Use this particular walk to get sunlight, see people, enjoy nature, pet a dog, and break a sweat. This kind of movement-and-pleasure-oriented walking has been shown to improve mood, increase functionality, decrease stress and anxiety, and even reduce pain.

Pace to Return to Work

Just as you can pace to get moving again, you can also pace to get back to work and resume your career. This is a useful strategy for increasing your ability to think, focus, and concentrate. If you haven't been able to do much work—reading, report-writing, strategizing—try this pacing plan to warm up your great brain! As with activity pacing, begin to pace for work by setting a specific, measurable goal. Then track the length of time you can comfortably read, write, or go to work on easy and tough days. Establish your daily baseline, and start pacing.

Here's how Percy paced:

Percy's Story

Percy had fibromyalgia and her body ached every day. She often felt dizzy and struggled with brain fog, making it hard to concentrate. She stopped going to work and was too fatigued to work from home. She had piles of reports to read. Just thinking about it made her body feel worse. She decided to try pacing with the support of her brother, who agreed to help motivate her by rewarding her for each step she took toward resuming work.

Percy's ultimate goal was to get through all of last month's reports. The amount of time she could read on a high-pain day was ten minutes. On a low-pain day, she could comfortably read for forty minutes. She completed her pacing worksheet and calculated a baseline daily reading time of twenty-three minutes.

Because complex, academic reports triggered stress and made pain worse, Percy decided to start pacing by reading a fun book. Each day, she set aside twenty-three minutes to read her enjoyable, relaxing book. Every day she read, her brother rewarded her with points. It felt simultaneously silly and nice to have such dedicated support, and the rewards and attention helped. Percy decided that, if she'd earned ten or more points by the end of the week, she'd put money aside for a trip to Hawaii.

The first week, it was hard for Percy to get herself to read when she was in pain. But she was motivated by thoughts of Hawaii. Percy added ten minutes of reading each week, even though some days were challenging. By month's end, she was reading two hours a day, taking tea breaks as needed, and feeling really proud. She slowly transitioned from pleasure-reading to reports, and within a month she was caught up.

Your Pacing Plan For Work

Step 1. Pick a work-related activity you'd like to resume (such as writing or going to the office).

_____

Step 2. State your ultimate goal for this activity using specific measurements like time, duration, and frequency.

_____

_____

Step 3. Measure the length of time (in minutes) you can do this activity comfortably on a low-pain day, then on a high-pain day.

Low-pain day: _____

High-pain day: _____

Step 4. Calculate the average by adding these times together, and then divide the total by two.

Low pain _____ + high pain _____ = _____ (total)

Total _____ ÷ 2 = _____ (average)

Step 5. Once you have an average amount of time you can do this activity, subtract a few minutes to give yourself a cushion. This will be your daily baseline: your goal whether it's a high- or low-pain day.

Average _____ − _____ minutes (cushion) = _____ (daily baseline)

Step 6. Plan to take a "rest and stretch" break after a set number of minutes, and establish the length of your break. This number will change from week to week as your strength and stamina increase.

Scheduled break every _____ number of minutes for _____ minutes.

Step 7. Each week, aim to add a few minutes to your activity, depending on tolerance, until you reach your goal.

Your weekly activity increase: _____ minutes

If your goal is to use pacing to resume work, make a plan to return gradually—even if it means starting with a few hours of work once a week. Work your way up to two half-days, then three. This will give your brain and body a chance to gradually adjust to the mental, physical, and social stimulation required to get through a work day. Like training for a marathon, pacing for chronic pain can help you achieve goals that might initially feel impossible.

Use this pacing worksheet to map out a week of pacing activities—walking, grocery shopping, swimming—and establish "active" and "rest" time goals. As you pace, remind yourself that it's okay to rest longer than intended, and to be active for less time than planned—especially at the beginning. Start wherever you can, and work your way up from there!

Weekly Pacing Plan

Activity	Goal Times (aspirational)	Actual Times						
		Mon.	Tues.	Wed.	Thurs.	Fri.	Sat.	Sun.
Walk	Active: 10 mins Rest: 5 mins	Active: 5 mins Rest: 10 mins	Active: 7 mins Rest: 11 mins	Active: 6 mins Rest: 8 mins	Active: 8 mins Rest: 10 mins	Active: 9 mins Rest: 7 mins	Active: 10 mins Rest: 6 mins	Active: 10 mins Rest: 6 mins
	Active: Rest:	Active: Rest:	Active: Rest:	Active: Rest:	Active: Rest:	Active: Rest:	Active: Rest:	Active: Rest:
	Active: Rest:	Active: Rest:	Active: Rest:	Active: Rest:	Active: Rest:	Active: Rest:	Active: Rest:	Active: Rest:
	Active: Rest:	Active: Rest:	Active: Rest:	Active: Rest:	Active: Rest:	Active: Rest:	Active: Rest:	Active: Rest:

You can find a blank Weekly Pacing Plan at http://www.newharbinger.com/46448.

Distraction Strategies

When you're absorbed in something fun, interesting, and distracting, pain can feel less bad. *Distraction strategies* help regulate pain by shifting attention away from pain and onto something else. Neuroscience reveals that when you're distracted, your prefrontal cortex (PFC, the frontmost part of your brain) sends a message to your pain dial, lowering pain volume. And when you tune in to and focus on pain, your PFC turns pain volume up.

Describe a time you were focusing on pain and noticed it started feeling worse:

_____

_____

Describe a time you were absorbed in a fun or interesting activity and noticed that pain seemed to fade into the background:

_____

_____

Distraction strategies can be *cognitive* (for the mind, like brain teasers), *physical* (activities, sensations, movements), or *emotional*. Like Malika, you can combine various types of distraction strategies to manage your pain.

Malika's Story

Malika lived with Lyme disease and constant joint pain. One Sunday afternoon, her friends got together to watch soccer—but Malika was stuck in bed with a flare-up. Her friends called repeatedly to encourage her to come over. Despite being in pain, she finally agreed, but became nervous in the car on the way over: What if her symptoms got worse after she left home? What if she was miserable and had to leave?

Once Malika arrived and saw her friends' smiling faces, she felt more at ease. They sat on the couch watching sports, eating pizza, and laughing. At the end of the game, Malika realized she'd been so distracted by fun activities (TV watching, being with friends), enjoyable sensations (lying on the soft sofa, savoring hot pizza, crunching chips, feeling seltzer fizzing on her tongue), and pleasant emotions (pleasure, happiness) that she hadn't noticed her symptoms for hours. Her pain wasn't gone, but it had become background noise.

Your Distraction Plan

Identify distraction strategies that might work for you so that you can start using them on tough days.

DISTRACT USING ACTIVITIES

Make a list of favorite activities and pick one—create art, write a story, go for a walk, cook a meal, play a game, watch golf, go shopping, or do something nice for someone (make a card for a friend, call your mom!). What activities distract you?

_____

_____

DISTRACT USING EMOTIONS

Read, watch, or listen to anything that generates pleasant emotions. Watch a funny movie, listen to a comedian, or read a comic book. Listen to a suspenseful podcast, read an interesting magazine, or watch a science program. Listen to calming songs or engage in a relaxing activity. Play an instrument and let the music move you. Notice how your mood changes when you change the situation. How can you distract yourself using emotions?

_____

_____

DISTRACT USING BRAIN TEASERS

Engage your brain with tasks that take your mind off pain. Try Sudoku or a crossword puzzle. Solve a book of riddles. Count backward from two hundred by sevens, list the presidents, or name all the constellations in the starry sky. Work on a complicated math problem or jigsaw puzzle. What mental exercises distract you?

_____

_____

DISTRACT USING YOUR FIVE SENSES

Use your five senses (sight, sound, taste, touch, and smell) to generate distracting sensations. Try cold or hot: apply ice to the back of your neck or give your feet a cold soak. Take a hot bath, light scented candles, listen to music, or drink something cool and soothing. Go for a walk outside at dusk and watch for bats. Get a massage. Which senses can you use to distract yourself?

_____

_____

Distraction Brainstorm

Here's a list of distraction strategies assembled by people similarly coping with pain and illness. Incorporate activities like the ones below into your daily pain-management routine. Check them off, cross them out, and add your own! In chapter 4 you'll find descriptions for strategies you may not be familiar with—for example, diaphragmatic breathing, guided meditation, and the body scan.

Take photos using a film camera.

Do a crossword puzzle.

Cook or bake.

Read.

Draw.

Write a story.

Practice diaphragmatic breathing.

Get fuzz therapy: pet your cat or dog.

Walk or bike around the block.

Go to the library and check out a book.

Hike in nature.

Head to a destination: the park, library, or corner mailbox to mail a letter.

Get coffee from the corner café.

See how many push-ups and sit-ups you can do.

Listen to a guided meditation.

Try Sudoku.

Play a board game.

Build something: a model airplane, a dog shed, or a new paper-towel holder for the kitchen.

Write a letter (a real letter, on paper!) to your niece, a friend, or a famous person.

Draw your family tree.

Ask the children in your life to help you make a list of the best Halloween costumes they've ever seen.

Video-chat with faraway friends or family members.

Go to a dog park and befriend someone else's dog.

List three goals you want to achieve, and one small step toward achieving each.

Listen to an audiobook.

Organize one corner of your room.

Run an errand.

Do laundry to enjoy the feeling of warm clothes fresh out of the dryer.

Try a biofeedback app.

Go to the grocery store and buy a fruit or vegetable you've never heard of before (what's a kumquat?).

Take a hot bath or cold shower.

Practice a body scan.

Try Five-Senses Mindfulness.

Identify species of flowers, birds, and butterflies outside using field guides.

Bounce a tennis ball against a wall.

Soak your feet in a bucket of ice water.

Self-soothe your five senses.

Write the story of how your parents met (ask them if you don't know!).

Look up adult classes, live or online, that sound interesting and register for one.

Color in a coloring book (such as a "zentangle" or mandala).

Research five places you'd like to visit.

Polish your nails or someone else's.

Think of all the types of (1) dogs, (2) cars, (3) TV shows, (4) sports, or (5) movies you can come up with.

Make a list of favorites: color, animal, season, food, TV show, movie, author, athlete, book, actor….

Look up your favorite recipe, write out the ingredients, and then make it.

Try guided imagery.

Stretch your muscles, one at a time.

Copy the words to a song, quote, or poem that makes you feel good and tape it to your wall.

Make up a dance.

Learn to crochet and make a hat for your godson.

List all the things you're looking forward to this week, big or small, as many as you can.

Invite friends over for a game of cards.

Ask a child—your son, niece, neighbor, or granddaughter—to tell you a story, and then write the ending together.

Make enough Rice Krispies treats to share with your entire family.

Add your own ideas here:

_____

_____

_____

_____

A Note About Screens

Screens can be useful tools for pain management. However, too much screen time can actually be harmful. Screens keep you sedentary and still, which prevents you from effectively desensitizing your pain system, and can contribute to the development and maintenance of chronic illness. Brains need exposure to real-life stimuli like people, movement, activity, and sunlight in order to heal.

Screens can also negatively impact sleep: Their blue light reduces the amount of *melatonin* (a sleep hormone) your brain produces. This delays feelings of sleepiness, makes it harder to fall asleep, and disrupts your natural sleep cycle. Screens also stimulate your brain, providing sensory overload during a time when you should be helping your brain slow down. Lastly, screens activate—rather than quiet—your nervous system, causing excitation rather than calm. (See chapter 7.)

Spending copious amounts of time on smartphones can also be stressful, despite the fact that we use them during our downtime. Increased time on screens and social media is associated with depression and anxiety, and can negatively impact self-esteem. A constant barrage of news reports, social media posts, emails, and other digital input activates the body's stress response—which can then amplify pain. Social media can also trigger self-criticism and negatively affect overall well-being.

In fact, research suggests that decreasing social media use can actually reduce stress, loneliness, and depression—which can then, in turn, lower pain volume. Consider going on a "social media diet" and temporarily delete social media apps for a few days, or take a break from your phone altogether by locking it away for twenty-four hours. Get some relief and give your brain a break. Try it: you might be surprised by how much you like it!

This doesn't mean you should avoid screens altogether—movies, TV shows, e-books, blogs, and videogames can serve as fun, helpful distractions. And social media can be a critical tool for connection, fostering community, and getting support. Just be aware of the amount of time you're on screens and know their drawbacks. Try to limit screen time to a few hours a day, and brainstorm other, non-screen activities that can reduce pain volume, like those on your distraction list.

Has social media or screen use ever made you feel stressed, sad, left out, or lonely? If so, when?

_____

_____

List two ways you can reduce your screen and social media use this week:

1. _____

2. _____

Soothe Your Senses

When you *self-soothe,* you comfort, take care of, and are kind to yourself. This is very important when you're chronically hurting. Self-soothing can turn off the false alarm signaling constant danger, inform your brain that your body is safe, and turn down the pain dial. To use this technique, consider how to best soothe each of your five senses: sight, sound, taste, touch, and smell. Combine these to make a *self-soothing plan* for tough days.

Sight: Walk in nature—the woods, the beach, a nearby park. Notice everything around you: the color of the trees and sky, the shapes of the clouds, the location of the sun in the sky. Paint. Draw. Print pictures of ocean vistas and hang them on your wall. Pick or buy a bouquet of colorful flowers for your room. Sit in a garden and watch butterflies, noticing their shape and flight. Watch your favorite movie. Drive to a lookout and admire the view. Stargaze.

What are your favorite things to look at?

_____

_____

Sound: Listen to relaxing, soothing music or your favorite musician. Listen to nature sounds, like rain, a waterfall, or your cat purring. Download the "Rain Rain" app or a white-noise app. Listen to an orchestra and pick out the different instruments. Tune in to a good music station or a YouTube video of a professional cellist. Go outside and listen to the wind in the trees. Hang a wind chime.

What are your favorite sounds?

_____

_____

Smell: Notice all the scents around you. Light a scented candle or incense. Take a shower with fragrant soap. Take walks in the woods, breathing in scents of nature. Smell every flower on your walk. Cook dinner and identify each scent. Visit a cosmetics store and sample all the perfumes. Try aromatherapy, especially lavender and eucalyptus. Bake cookies!

What are the most soothing scents?

_____

_____

Taste: Make "comfort food" or a favorite meal, and notice how the taste soothes you. Eat slowly, savoring each bite. Tune in to temperature and textures. Drink a mug of hot tea with honey. Make your grandmother's chicken soup and sip it slowly, feeling it soothe your throat and belly. Crunch on ice, or drink a cold glass of lemonade. Pop a cold, crunchy grape in your mouth.

What are the most soothing things to taste?

_____

_____

Touch: Notice textures, temperatures, and sensations. Take a warm bubble bath, or soak in a hot tub. Rub an ice cube on your neck. Cuddle with your partner, child, dog, or cat and notice how comforted you feel. Hold someone's hand. Ask for a hug. Pop bubble wrap. Put on your favorite cozy pajamas or an oversized sweatshirt. Hold a heating pad on the spot that hurts. Wrap yourself in fuzzy blankets; try a weighted blanket.

What are the most comforting sensations?

_____

_____

Put all these together to make a self-soothing plan for tough days. A good self-soothing plan, like Juliana's, incorporates all five of your senses to maximally soothe both brain and body.

Juliana's Story

Juliana was having a tough day and her whole body hurt. To soothe, she made a plan using each of her five senses. She ran hot water for a bath (touch). She used a "bath bomb," which releases a scent, bubbles, fizzes, and turns the water pink (smell, sight). She gathered colorful magazines with pictures and distracting stories (sight). She poured a tall glass of iced tea because she liked contrasting the hot water on her skin with a cold drink (taste, touch). She played her favorite playlist (sound). As Juliana sank into the bath, she focused on her soothed senses. For the entire hour she was submerged, she felt relaxed and peaceful. When she got out, Juliana said to her sister, "I feel like a new woman!"

Write your own five-senses self-soothing plan here:

_____

_____

_____

_____

_____

_____

Scheduling Pleasurable Activities

Living with pain or illness can mean giving up things you love, like favorite hobbies and activities. But this only makes you feel worse, because you experience less pleasure. When you have pain, it's even *more* important to schedule activities that give you joy! Every minute you're engaged in a pleasurable activity is a minute you're less stressed, sad, and focused on pain. Moreover, pleasurable activities can increase levels of neurotransmitters like serotonin (regulates mood), endorphins (natural painkillers), and dopamine (regulates feelings of reward and pleasure). These neurochemicals can then turn down your pain dial.

What are some activities that give you pleasure? (Circle any that apply and add your own.)

Cooking	Drawing	Baking bread
Karate	Hanging out with friends	Playing drums
Cheese-making	Designing clothes	Camping
Bowling	Acting in plays	Going to concerts
Singing	Ballroom dancing	Woodworking
Football	Tennis	Horseback riding
Bubble baths	Swimming	Playing chess
Fishing	Playing catch with the dog	_____
Mahjong	Making pottery	_____

Integrate pleasurable activities into daily life so that you make sure to do something enjoyable every single day. This is *especially* important on days you have pain. Schedule one pleasurable activity every day this week. Make sure to specify time and place (*e.g., Monday: walk to the turtle pond at 9 a.m.*):

Monday: _____

Tuesday: _____

Wednesday: _____

Thursday: _____

Friday: _____

Saturday: _____

Sunday: _____

How can you make sure to incorporate pleasurable activities into your daily life? (*e.g., Block off "turtle-time" in my calendar*)

_____

_____

Two Steps Forward...

Anyone with chronic pain—and anyone treating it—will tell you that progress is often "two steps forward, one step back." The process of treating chronic pain typically involves some progress...then a pain flare...then more work, more progress...then another flare. It can be frustrating, aggravating, and discouraging. But it's critical that you not give up hope. When hope goes, motivation goes with it! For this reason, it's important to plan ahead as you work your way through this book. Be familiar with the forward-backward-forward process, manage expectations, anticipate setbacks, and be prepared. Feeling prepared can reduce fear and frustration. In chapter 8 you'll put together a Pain Plan so that you know exactly what to do in case of a flare. By the end of this book, your plan will be loaded with helpful tools and strategies. Start adding ideas to your plan now so that you can be more confident in the face of pain.

Name a time in your life you experienced this "two-steps-forward-one-step-back" phenomenon:

_____

_____

How did you make it through?

_____

_____

_____

What's one thing you'll say to yourself during a flare to help you keep going? (*e.g., A flare doesn't mean my Pain Plan isn't working. I've survived 800 flares and I can get through this one!*)

_____

_____

Conclusion

Pain and illness can keep you sedentary, stuck, and miserable. While it's instinctive to stop all activity, rest, and self-protect in the face of pain, avoiding and withdrawing only sensitize brain and body, amplifying chronic pain. One way to fight back is to work backward, set goals, and pace to gradually resume physical activities, social activities, work, pleasurable activities, and hobbies you love. You can also turn down pain volume by distracting and soothing your (always connected!) brain and body.

In the next chapter, you'll learn mind-body medicine tools like relaxation strategies, mindfulness, and biofeedback to help control pain.

CHAPTER 4

Mind-Body Medicine

There's no getting around it: your brain and body are connected 100% of the time. Biopsychosocial forces work together to control your pain dial, turning pain volume up and down. *Mind-body medicine* uses the power of your brain to alter neurochemistry, turn off the danger alarm, and take charge of pain. Research shows that these strategies—which include relaxation, mindfulness, biofeedback, and imagery—can decrease pain frequency and intensity, increase control over physical symptoms, reduce negative emotions like sadness and stress, and increase quality of life. Mind-body techniques can also alter major bodily functions like muscle tension, heart rate, skin temperature, and immune functioning. Imagine the power you'd possess if you could use your brain to help heal your body!

In this chapter you'll learn a variety of mind-body medicine strategies including Diaphragmatic Breathing, Body Scan, and Five-Senses Mindfulness to rewire your pain system, facilitate feelings of safety and calm, and lower pain volume. If pain levels don't change right away, that's okay—try to stick with it, practicing a little bit every day. The more you practice pain-mastery skills, the bigger and stronger the brain's "pain-mastery pathway" will become. The stronger this pathway gets, the better you'll get at changing your pain. Think of it as taking daily pain medicine!

Relaxation Strategies

Relaxation strategies, which are central to evidence-based treatments like cognitive behavioral therapy (CBT) and mindfulness-based stress reduction (MBSR), affect your *physiology*—the physical and biochemical processes that underlie health, pain, and functioning. These strategies can be used to decrease stress, anxiety, muscle tension, and blood pressure; alter brain chemistry; increase blood flow for faster healing; slow heart rate; change hormone and neurotransmitter levels; improve sleep; help you feel more in control of your body; and lower the pain dial. They can also give you greater capacity to cope with pain, symptoms, and whatever else life throws your way.

Try practicing relaxation strategies when pain is medium to low rather than during an intense flare. It's easier to learn new skills when you're not distressed. Then, once you've mastered them, you can apply them to the difficult situations that require them most.

Diaphragmatic Breathing

Relaxation strategies often start with diaphragmatic, or belly, breathing. Your *diaphragm* is a muscle just below your ribs that contracts and expands when you breathe. Most of us tend to chest breathe, especially when we're stressed, sick, or in pain. This shallow chest breathing provides less oxygen to your brain and can make you feel dizzy, lightheaded, or faint. It also keeps your SNS activated and your pain system sensitive. Test to see if you're chest breathing by putting a hand on your chest and see if it rises when you inhale.

In contrast, relaxed diaphragmatic breathing uses your diaphragm and stomach muscles. When you belly breathe, you train your breath to go lower and slower. This increases your blood oxygen level, improves circulation to facilitate healing, lowers stress hormones like cortisol and adrenaline, turns off your SNS to calm your body, and helps reduce pain volume.

Check which type of breathing you're doing—stressed versus relaxed—throughout the day, and catch yourself when your breathing gets stressed and shallow. The moment you notice that you're chest breathing is the moment you can change your physiology, shut off your SNS stress response, and lower your pain dial by breathing lower and slower instead.

HOW TO DO IT

Set aside five minutes for this activity. You can download a recording of this exercise at http://www.newharbinger.com/46448 or ask someone to read it to you.

Check in with your body and emotions:

Pain rating on a scale from 0 to 10 (0 = none, 5 = moderate, 10 = severe): _____

Stress or anxiety level on a scale from 0 to 10 (0 = none, 5 = moderate, 10 = extreme): _____

Find a quiet place where you won't be disturbed. Turn off your screens and put them away. Set a timer for five minutes. Lie or sit somewhere comfortable and quiet, like the couch. Uncross your arms and legs and close your eyes. Place one hand on your belly and the other hand on your chest.

Remind yourself that, in this moment, you have nowhere to go and nothing else to do. Tell yourself that you're safe.

Imagine your attention is a spotlight and you can control where it shines.

Focus the spotlight of attention on your breath.

Take a slow, deep breath in.

Notice how the air feels at your nose, and how it feels going down into your lungs.

Slowly exhale.

On your next inhale, send the breath down into your belly.

Feel your belly expand as if it's a balloon. Feel the hand on your belly rise.

If the hand on your chest moves when you breathe in, send the air lower, into your belly.

Hold your breath for a moment, and notice your belly, full of air. Notice the urge to exhale.

Then release the breath slowly. As you exhale, let your shoulders drop and your back relax. Feel your stomach muscles relax. Notice your hand lowering as the air leaves your body.

Take another breath in. Focus all your attention just on your breath. Let your breathing be low and slow.

With each in-breath, send the air all the way down into your belly. With each out-breath, say "Relax" to yourself, and imagine all the tension draining out of your body.

Do this until the timer rings. If your mind wanders, gently bring the spotlight of attention back to your breath.

Check in with your body and emotions:

New stress or anxiety rating on a scale from 0 to 10 (0 = none, 5 = moderate, 10 = extreme): _____

New pain rating on a scale from 0 to 10 (0 = none, 5 = moderate, 10 = severe): _____

What did you notice about your body? Your emotions?

_____

_____

_____

Plan to practice this at a set time every day this week (*Example: Mornings at 7 a.m.*):

_____

How will you remember to practice? (*Example: Leave a note for myself on the breakfast table*)

_____

Body Scan

In your brain there lives a map of your entire body called the *homunculus*. This neurological map contains sensory and motor information about your body, forming a mini-body map. If, for example, you sense into your left foot, noticing how it feels (sensation) and what it's doing (movement), you're activating your homunculus!

The *body scan* is a technique that uses this brain map along with mindfulness, relaxation, and *somatic* (body) awareness to change pain. It can help you regulate attention and tune in to muscle tension and stress, and it offers the opportunity to observe your body from the inside out. As you go through the body, you may feel intense sensations, subtle sensations, or nothing at all. You may also discover areas that are tense and tight. If you can let the tension go and allow your muscles to soften, do so. However, if you can't, that's also okay. There's no need to strive for any particular outcome. You may also notice that your mind wants to think, worry, and plan. This is normal. Just let all thoughts and sensations be, noticing how they feel, how they change, and what emotions they bring with them.

HOW TO DO IT

Set aside ten to fifteen minutes for this activity. You can download a recording of this exercise at http://www.newharbinger.com/46448 or have someone read it to you.

Check in with your body and emotions:

Pain rating on a scale from 0 to 10 (0 = none, 5 = moderate, 10 = severe): _____

Stress or anxiety level on a scale from 0 to 10 (0 = none, 5 = moderate, 10 = extreme): _____

Find a quiet place where you won't be disturbed. Turn off your screens and put them away. Lie somewhere comfortable and quiet, like the couch or the floor. Use a blanket to keep your body warm. Uncross your arms and legs and close your eyes.

Place one hand on your chest and the other on your belly.

Take in a slow, deep belly breath.

Focus the spotlight of attention on the air as it travels in through your nose.

Notice whether the air is warm or cool, and how it tickles the inside of your nose.

On your next in-breath, feel the air travel down into your belly. Feel your belly expand like a balloon as you inhale; feel the hand on your belly rise. Hold the breath for a moment. When you exhale, release the breath slowly. Feel the air at your nose as you breathe out, and notice whether it's warm or cool. Let all of your breaths be belly breaths.

Now send your attention down to your feet. Feel your feet in your shoes, and notice the fabric of your socks on your skin. Feel your heels resting on the couch. Notice whether your feet are warm or cool. If there's any tension in your feet, see if you can let that tension go. If not, just let the sensations be.

Sense up into your ankles, shins, and calf muscles. Feel the backs of your calves on the couch or floor. Feel the fabric of your pants on your skin. Notice whether your shins are warm or cool. If there's any tension in your lower legs, shins, or calves, see if you can let that tension go. If not, just let the sensations be.

Sense into your upper legs, thighs, quads, and hamstrings. Feel the fabric of your pants on your legs. Notice the backs of your thighs on the couch. Notice whether your upper legs are warm or cool. If there's any tension in your thighs, quads, or hamstrings, see if you can let that tension go. Let your legs be heavy…limp…loose…and relaxed. Imagine that they're melting into the couch.

Sense into your hips and up into your belly. Feel your hand resting on your belly, and notice the warmth there. Feel your belly fill with air as you breathe in…and feel your stomach muscles relax as you slowly breathe out. Sense into your stomach and notice whether you're hungry or full, and if your stomach is making any sounds. Without any judgment, just observe. If there's any tension in your stomach or intestines, see if you can let that tension go. Allow your stomach and intestines to completely relax and unwind.

Sense into your chest, heart, and lungs. Notice your pulse as your heart pumps blood around your body. Feel your warm hand on your chest. Notice your lungs expand when you breathe in…and feel them relax when you breathe out. If there's any tension in your chest, heart, or lungs, see if you can let that tension go.

Send your attention up to your shoulders. Let your shoulders slump, as if gravity is pulling them down. Sense into your arms, noticing whether your skin is warm or cool. Feel the fabric of your shirt on your skin. Let relaxation flow from the top of your shoulders, past your elbows, down into your forearms, wrists, and hands, all the way down into your palms and fingertips. Feel your warm hands on your chest and belly. If there's any tension in your shoulders, arms, hands, or fingers, just let that tension go. Let your arms be heavy…limp…loose…and relaxed.

Sense into your back. Feel the couch against your back, and notice how you're held and supported. Notice your upper back, middle back, lower back. Feel the fabric of your shirt on your skin. Notice whether your back is warm or cool. If there's any tension in your upper, middle, or lower back, see if you can let that tension go. Notice all sensations, thoughts, and emotions.

Send your attention up your neck and around to the back of your head. Feel your head supported by the couch. Notice where your head touches the pillow; feel your hair on your neck and scalp. Notice whether your neck and head are warm or cool. If there's any tension in your neck, let that tension go. Sense into your temples and release any tension. Allow your neck and head to feel heavy and relaxed.

Send your attention down to the muscles of your face. Notice your facial expression. Sense into your forehead, temples, eyebrows. Feel your eyes behind your eyelids. Sense into your cheeks and jaw muscles, and let your jaw hang open as it relaxes. Sense into your mouth and notice your tongue. If there's any tension anywhere in your face, let that tension go. Allow all your muscles to be limp, loose, and soft.

Sense into your ears and notice everything you can hear. Take a moment to just listen. Make a mental list of all the sounds you hear without any judgment. If you start thinking about other things, gently bring your attention back to your ears.

Now do a full scan of your body, from the top of your head, down your neck, into your chest and back, down your shoulders and arms, stomach and hips, legs, past your knees, all the way down to your toes. Feel your entire body as a whole, noticing all sensations, thoughts, and emotions. Notice how relaxed and calm you feel. This is your safe place. You carry it inside of you, and you can come back here whenever you choose.

Now, with eyes still closed, picture the room you're in. Imagine the walls and furniture. Wiggle your fingers and toes, and when you're ready, slowly open your eyes.

Check in with your body and emotions:

New stress or anxiety rating on a scale from 0 to 10 (0 = none, 5 = moderate, 10 = extreme): _____

New pain rating on a scale from 0 to 10 (0 = none, 5 = moderate, 10 = severe): _____

What did you notice physically and emotionally? Were there any surprising sensations? Where did you discover tension?

_____

_____

_____

Schedule a time to practice this once daily, specifying time and place (*Example: At the office at 4 p.m.*):

_____

Pocket Relaxation

Now that you have the power to relax mind and body, here's a one-minute "pocket" relaxation to take with you wherever you go. Carry it in your pocket to use at work, the hospital, the grocery store, when you're stuck in traffic, or anytime you have a pain flare. No one needs to know you're doing it. It can help you catch stress, pain, and tension before they get too intense, and takes only a minute to do.

HOW TO DO IT

Find a place for a private time-out, or simply stay where you are. Close your eyes if that feels comfortable, and place one hand on your belly. Take a deep belly breath. Hold it for a few seconds and feel it in your body. Now *slowly* exhale, and say "*Relax*" to yourself. Let your whole body relax: from the top of your head...face...neck and shoulders...arms...hands...upper and lower back... around to your chest...your stomach...hips and thighs...knees...calves...all the way down to your toes. Let your body get limp, heavy, and loose, like a wet noodle. Imagine stress and pain draining out of your body like a liquid, flowing out of your feet and down into the ground. Hold that relaxed feeling and slowly count to twenty. Then slowly open your eyes. Remember—the more you use this skill, the better you'll get at it! Try it a few times a day and see how you feel.

Jay's Story

Jay runs a successful company. He's had terrible back pain for years and often has flare-ups at work. When this happens, Jay goes into the break room, lies down on the conference table, closes his eyes, and uses his mind to scan his whole body, head to toe. He relaxes every tense muscle, paying particular attention to his back. He releases stored stress slowly, vertebra by vertebra. He imagines the stress and tension flowing out of his body like black ink, running down the table legs and sinking down into the ground. This helps him relax and feel more in control of pain, and allows him to finish his workday.

Write down your own ideas for times to use this pocket relaxation (*Examples: At my son's hockey game; in the doctor's waiting room; before bed*):

1. _____

2. _____

3. _____

Progressive Muscle Relaxation

Muscle tension is common when we have pain because our bodies normally and naturally tense, tighten, and brace in response to painful stimuli. While this may seem like a good way to "prepare" for pain, research shows that bracing and tension actually make pain worse. Daily stress, frustration, and anger can further increase muscle tension and pain. *Progressive muscle relaxation* (PMR) helps you cultivate bodily awareness so that you can catch and release stress and tension before they trigger or exacerbate pain. While doing this exercise, be gentle with the parts of your body that hurt. You can skip body parts as needed.

HOW TO DO IT

Set aside ten to fifteen minutes for this activity. You can download a recording of this exercise at http://www.newharbinger.com/46448 or have someone read it to you.

Check in with your body and emotions:

Pain rating on a scale from 0 to 10 (0 = none, 5 = moderate, 10 = severe): _____

Stress or anxiety level on a scale from 0 to 10 (0 = none, 5 = moderate, 10 = extreme): _____

Find a quiet place where you won't be disturbed. Turn off your screens and put them away. Sit somewhere comfortable and quiet, like the couch.

During this exercise, you will tense and release various muscle groups one at a time, paying extra attention to the difference between how it feels when muscles are tense and tight, and how it feels when they're loose and relaxed.

Start with your feet. Flex them by pulling your toes up toward the sky while pressing your heels into the floor. Notice the tension in your foot muscles, and count to ten. Let go of the tension in your foot muscles and let them relax. Notice the flow of relaxation and warmth as your muscles relax.

Move your attention up to your calf muscles. Contract them by lifting the heels of your feet off the floor while pressing your toes into the ground. Feel the tension in your calves and hold this position for ten seconds. Press harder into the ground to increase tension. When you reach the count of ten, let your heels drop and release the tension. Notice the flow of warmth and relaxation in your calves.

Move your attention to your knees and thighs. Extend your legs out straight and tense your thigh muscles. Press your thighs and knees together and squeeze tightly. Hold this tension in your upper legs and continue squeezing for a count of ten. Then exhale and release all the tension in your upper legs. Feel the warmth and relaxation in your thighs.

Move your attention up to your stomach muscles. Tense your abdomen by sucking it in and clenching the muscles. Squeeze harder, then even harder. Hold this tension in your stomach for a count of ten, then relax and release the muscles. Feel the warmth and relaxation spread through your stomach.

Move your attention up to your shoulders, lifting them up to your ears. Hold your shoulders tight for a count of ten—raise them high, then even higher. Now release the muscles and let them just drop and relax. Feel gravity pulling them down, and notice the flow of relaxation as your shoulders relax.

Tense your bicep muscles by making a fist, then bringing your fist toward your shoulder and tightening your biceps. Count to ten while squeezing tighter and tighter. Then release your biceps and let your arms fall to your side. Feel the blood rush down your arms into your hands as your muscles relax.

Now clench your hands into fists, and squeeze them tightly for ten seconds. Focus on the sensations in your hand and notice how tight the muscles are. Then release the muscles and let your hands hang limp and loose. Notice how warm and relaxed they feel.

Send your attention up your neck and into your face. Tense your facial muscles by clenching your teeth and tensing the muscles in your jaw, wrinkling your nose and squeezing your eyes shut. Raise your eyebrows and tense the muscles in your forehead. Tense all the muscles in your face, and hold this position for a count of ten. Then release all the muscles in your face and let your jaw hang open. Notice the difference.

Now do a scan of your whole body. Feel the relaxation flow from the top of your head, down into your face, down into your neck and shoulders, down your arms into your hands, into your chest, down into your stomach, past your hips, down into your thighs and knees, down into your calves and shins, past your ankles, and all the way down into your feet. Notice how heavy, still, and relaxed your body feels. Let the feeling of relaxation spread through your entire body. Remind yourself that you can come back to this safe, relaxed place whenever you like.

Check in with your body and emotions:

New stress or anxiety rating on a scale from 0 to 10 (0 = none, 5 = moderate, 10 = extreme): _____

New pain rating on a scale from 0 to 10 (0 = none, 5 = moderate, 10 = severe): _____

Schedule a time to practice this week (*Example: Friday at 4 p.m.*):

_____   _____

How will you remember to use PMR this week? (*Example: Set a timer on my phone*)

_____

Mindfulness

Mindfulness techniques are an integral part of many chronic-pain treatments, and have a robust research base. *Mindfulness* is the quality or state of being present, attuned, and self-aware; of letting your experience, whatever it is, just unfold without any judgment or criticism. Mindfulness emphasizes noticing things exactly as they are, without trying to push them away or change them. It's the state that arises when you stop forcing yourself to feel, or not feel, any particular way—when you stop trying to beat pain out of existence, stop fighting pain, and instead allow all sensations to just be. While it's natural and normal to want to get rid of pain, it simply isn't always possible. Sometimes the best we can do is drop the battle and learn to coexist. Mindfulness can help with this difficult task.

When we are mindful, we use our brain's "attention muscle" to focus on what's happening inside us and around us in the present moment without judging anything as "good" or "bad." This can be challenging, because our minds naturally tend to drift backward into the past: *I shouldn't have done that!* Or, *Why did I say that? That was so stupid!* Lying in bed at the end of a long day, it's natural to take account of events, mistakes, and regrets. But focusing on the past can be stressful, because these things have already happened and we can't do much about them.

Our minds also tend to shoot forward into the future: *What's going to happen to me? What if I never get better? What if things get worse?* Ruminating about the future is anxiety-provoking because we can't predict or control it, no matter how hard we try. This stress only turns up the pain dial and makes pain even worse.

Mindfulness is the muscle we use to pull our attention from the past (what's behind us) and from the future (what's in front of us) back into the present moment. *Just right here.* Because chances are, you can handle Just Right Here. Here you are, sitting in a chair, reading this book. And you can manage this moment.

Mindfulness can also change unhelpful responses to triggering situations and events by inserting a pause between trigger and response, giving us the freedom to intentionally choose new, more effective responses. This includes altering instinctive responses to pain such as tensing, guarding, bracing, and avoiding.

Mindfulness Changes the Pain Response

	Old Pattern	New Pattern
Trigger	Leg pain	Leg pain
Mindfulness?	No	Yes
Response	Clench leg muscles, brace against pain, get angry and frustrated.	Pause, breathe, massage leg, allow leg muscles to relax, stop fighting.

One mindfulness-based approach to pain management is MBSR, a scientifically-supported intervention for chronic pain that integrates mindfulness and relaxation strategies to calm the mind, relax the body, change brain activation, and lower pain volume. In addition to investigating pain and tension in the body, MBSR allows us to work with the uncomfortable emotions that naturally come with chronic pain—validating, acknowledging, and allowing them to be rather than resisting or judging them. This can help us expand our ability to be with pain one moment at a time.

The Neurobiology of Mindfulness

While mindfulness is something we *do*, it also affects how we *think* and *feel*. Regular mindfulness practice can decrease distress and disability, improve concentration and sleep, improve quality of life, increase ability to manage and cope with pain, and decrease intensity and frequency of pain flares.

How does mindfulness change pain? Neuroscience provides some answers. In addition to physiological changes in the body—reduced muscle tension, lower blood pressure, slower heart rate—mindfulness also changes the *brain*. Studies suggest that mindfulness may decrease pain-related activity in the prefrontal cortex, a brain region involved in pain regulation. Mindfulness may also effect change via increased activity in the anterior cingulate cortex and the anterior insula, brain regions involved in the emotional and cognitive components of pain. Because your brain is *plastic*— flexible and ever-changing—the brain's "mindfulness muscle" gets bigger and stronger the more you use it!

While mindfulness isn't a magic cure, some people with chronic pain report remarkable results. Here's Arun's experience:

Arun's Story

Arun had beaten cancer twice. The disease and its treatment were physically and emotionally grueling, and he worried about a relapse. After two years in remission, he came home after a basketball game with excruciating pain shooting from his lower back to his feet. His doctor ordered an MRI and diagnosed him with degenerative disc disease. Over the next three years, Arun tried many interventions, including physical therapy, massage, and medications. Nothing helped. The pain got worse, spreading to his legs, neck, and shoulders. It got so bad that he relegated himself to bed, declining all invitations and activities. Arun sank into a deep depression. His orthopedist suggested surgery, but after surviving cancer he didn't want any more procedures. Arun took matters into his own hands, reading everything he could about pain, and discovered research on mindfulness. He was skeptical, but felt he had nothing to lose. While meditating and practicing body scans, his pain started to move and change. As pain decreased, he was able to tune in to his triggers: a stressful job, perfectionism, and unprocessed trauma from his cancer diagnosis. He committed to regular practice, registered for mindfulness retreats, changed his job, decreased stress, and began to effectively manage his pain. He's resumed basketball, work, and social activities, and is living his life. Pain is no longer in charge and he has learned how to coexist with it.

Practicing Mindfulness

The practice of mindfulness typically involves the following steps:

1. Go inside yourself, get quiet, and tune in. Focus your attention on breath and body.

2. Notice when your attention wanders. Label what your mind is doing without judgment or self-criticism (thinking, planning, daydreaming, worrying).

3. Gently bring your attention back to your breath, body, and the present moment.

The real challenge often isn't learning mindfulness—it's setting aside the time to practice it. In this chapter you'll learn a variety of mindfulness techniques and how to integrate these strategies into your daily life.

Watching the Breath

One effective way to invite your mind into the present moment is to focus on your breath. Your breath is always with you. It's constant and calming, like waves in the sea. Focusing on your breath pulls your attention into your body so that you can be in the here and now.

HOW TO DO IT

Set aside five minutes for this activity.

Before you start, check in with your body and emotions:

Pain rating on a scale from 0 to 10 (0 = none, 5 = moderate, 10 = severe): _____

Stress or anxiety rating on a scale from 0 to 10 (0 = none, 5 = moderate, 10 = extreme): _____

Mindful check-in: What situations or events from this week were triggering, stressful, or upsetting?

_____

_____

What emotions are you feeling in this moment?

_____

_____

Find a quiet place where you won't be disturbed. Turn off your screens and put them away. Lie or sit somewhere comfortable and quiet, like the couch. Uncross your arms and legs and close your eyes.

Imagine that your attention is a spotlight and you can control where it shines.

Shine that spotlight on your breath as it comes in through your nose.

Examine this in-breath with curiosity, as if you've never noticed how air feels before.

Without any judgment, feel the air tickle the inside of your nose.

Notice whether the air is warm or cool.

On your next in-breath, notice how the air feels traveling down into your lungs.

Feel your lungs expand and stretch as air comes into your body. Notice how your chest rises.

Hold your breath for a moment, noticing how it feels.

Notice the urge to release your breath.

Now gently exhale, feeling your lungs relax and your chest fall as the air leaves your body.

Notice the sound of your out-breath.

Notice the muscles in your body relax as you exhale.

Feel the air at your nose, noticing how it tickles the inside of your nose.

Notice whether the air is warm or cool.

No need to do or change anything; just notice how your body feels when you breathe.

Now bring that spotlight of attention to your ears.

Notice, in this quiet moment, what sounds you can hear. Try not to judge sounds as good or bad—just observe and report, like a forecaster reporting the weather.

If your mind starts to wander, that's okay. Simply bring that spotlight of attention back to your breath.

If you noticed thoughts intruding or your mind bouncing, that's okay—it's your mind's job to think. All you need do is simply notice when attention wanders, and gently bring it back again to your breath. If you have trouble concentrating during these practices, try keeping a running, internal commentary of everything you notice while sitting. "I feel my feet on the ground, I feel my legs touching the chair, I feel the air in my lungs, I hear the sound of my exhale." This will help ground you in the present moment.

Check in with your body and emotions:

New stress or anxiety rating on a scale from 0 to 10 (0 = none, 5 = moderate, 10 = extreme): _____

New pain rating on a scale from 0 to 10 (0 = none, 5 = moderate, 10 = severe): _____

What did you notice and how did you feel, emotionally and physically?

_____

_____

_____

When and where can you practice mindfulness? Note time and place. (*Example: At work I can practice at my desk during lunchtime; at home I can practice in my living room nightly at 9 p.m.*)

At home: _____

_____

At work: _____

_____

Schedule a time to practice this week, specifying time and place (*Example: 7 a.m. on the couch before breakfast*):

_____

How will you remember to use this tool this week? (*Example: Set a timer on my phone*)

_____

Mindfulness of Change

An important aspect of mindfulness, particularly for chronic pain, is allowing yourself, despite all instincts to the contrary, to be present with bodily sensations and emotions without pushing them away or judging them as awful. This practice can expand your tolerance of difficult sensations and emotions. It can also allow you to experience pain differently—increasing your awareness of the ever-changing nature of pain, transforming your relationship with pain, and allowing you to be with it in a new way. Rather than loathing, hating, and attempting to excise pain, this practice can enable you to observe it more objectively, like a weather forecaster reporting the weather. Some people report that creating this distance enables them to notice things they didn't notice before: the color, size, and shape of their pain; the way it moves, morphs, and changes as they sit with it; and the way it ebbs and flows. Moreover, reducing the amount of time spent battling and fighting with pain—and failing—can reduce your misery and suffering.

Cathy's Story

After sustaining a running injury, Cathy developed complex regional pain syndrome (CRPS) in her right leg. After countless appointments and procedures failed to cure her pain, she registered for an MBSR class. Cathy noticed that constantly fighting her pain—attempting to vanquish and destroy it—caused anger, frustration, and suffering. Through regular, daily mindfulness practice, she learned to increase her tolerance of just sitting with her pain—walking with it, sleeping with it, even embracing it. She described her new relationship with pain as "walking a dog on a leash." Like a puppy, her pain required some care and management, but she accepted that it was part of her life and was likely going to be with her for a while. She noticed that the instant she stopped fighting and struggling with her pain, it started feeling less bad.

Use the mindful check-in below to become an "internal investigator," quietly looking inside your body without doing, fighting with, or changing anything. Observe thoughts, emotions, and physical sensations just as you'd watch clouds drift across the sky.

HOW TO DO IT

Set aside five minutes for this activity. You can download a recording of this exercise at http://www.newharbinger.com/46448 or ask someone to read it to you.

Find a quiet place where you won't be disturbed. Turn off your screens and put them away. Lie somewhere comfortable and quiet, like the couch. Uncross your arms and legs and close your eyes.

Focus the spotlight of attention on your breath.

Remind yourself that, in this peaceful moment, you have nowhere to be and nothing else to do.

Remind yourself that you are safe.

Take a slow, deep breath in.

Notice how the air feels at your nose. Notice whether it's warm or cool, and how it feels going down into your belly.

As you breathe in, feel your belly expand as if it's a balloon. Hold the breath for a moment and notice your belly, full of air. Notice the urge to exhale.

Then release the breath. As you exhale, notice your shoulders drop and your back relax. Feel your stomach muscles relax. Feel the air at your nose, and notice whether it's warm or cool.

Focus all your attention just on your breath. Let your breathing be low and slow.

Now allow yourself to sense into the place that hurts. Let your attention rest lightly on the place of pain.

Without any judgment, describe your pain. Describe its color, shape, temperature, texture, and location.

Hold your attention there, without pushing the pain away or avoiding the sensations.

Examine, explore, and observe.

Notice, as you lie here, how your pain changes. Notice if it moves, changes shape or color, switches from hot to cold, expands or contracts. Be present with all the sensations in your body.

Allow the pain to just be.

Notice thoughts as they arrive. Without pushing them away, simply watch them, like clouds in the sky.

Sense into your emotions. Notice how you feel. Label each emotion and then let it go, like a colorful balloon.

Now move your attention to your hands and arms. Gently stroke your arms with your fingertips. Focus completely on the sensation of soothing touch.

With eyes still closed, picture the room you're in, the walls and furniture. Wiggle your fingers and toes, and when you're ready, slowly open your eyes.

What did you notice about your body that you hadn't noticed before?

_____

_____

Describe how your pain changed over the course of this practice. Note changes in location, size, shape, color, and temperature:

_____

_____

What thoughts and emotions arose? What was it like to sit with them?

_____

_____

Schedule a time and place to practice this week (*Example: Tomorrow at noon on the couch*):

_____

How will you remember to use this tool this week? (*Example: Write it on my calendar*)

_____

Five-Senses Mindfulness

You can also strengthen your mindfulness muscle by tuning into your five senses. Your powers of perception are always working whether you're attuned to them or not. Practice being "in the moment" by mindfully experiencing your senses of sight, sound, touch, taste, and smell. The Five-Senses Mindfulness exercise can decrease stress and frustration, increase joy and pleasure, alter the flow of attention, and promote relaxation. Use this strategy to ground, calm, and soothe yourself anytime you're feeling stressed or having a pain flare.

HOW TO DO IT

Set aside ten minutes for this activity.

Check in with your body and emotions:

Pain rating on a scale from 0 to 10 (0 = none, 5 = moderate, 10 = severe): _____

Stress or anxiety level on a scale from 0 to 10 (0 = none, 5 = moderate, 10 = extreme): _____

Select a piece of fruit from your kitchen (you'll need it for "taste") and go outside. Find a spot in your yard or a park where you won't be disturbed. If you can't go outside, select a favorite room in your house. Turn off your screens. Practice diaphragmatic breathing, letting your breathing be slow and relaxed.

Sight: If you're outside, focus on the nature around you. Use your eyes to scan your surroundings. Notice shapes, shadows, and textures. Notice colors: green, white, yellow. How many different flowers and trees do you see? Look up at the sky and describe the colors. Notice the clouds. Where's the sun? If you're inside, describe the room: furniture, colors, textures. Describe the quality of light, number of chairs, sofa fabric, shapes in the ceiling. Without any judgment, describe everything you see.

Sound: Close your eyes, tune in to your ears, and notice everything you hear. If you're inside, and can't go out, open a window. Tune in to the sound of the wind in the trees, the birds singing. Notice cars in the distance, dogs barking, children playing. Listen to music playing, or rain on the pavement. What can you hear?

Touch: Rub your fingers along different surfaces and textures. If you're outside, touch a leaf, flower petal, tree trunk, park bench. Feel the sun on your skin and the breeze in your hair. If you're inside, find different textures and temperatures—smooth, rough, bumpy, cold, warm—and describe them. Feel the cool metal of the teakettle, the softness of the carpet, the texture of your favorite blanket. Take a step and notice your feet in your shoes. What can you feel?

Smell: Breathe deeply. Notice everything you smell. If you're outdoors, find a fragrant plant or tree, smell a flower, rub a blade of grass between your fingers. If you're inside, explore different scents in your home: open a jar of cinnamon, sample perfume, rub mint leaves in your palm, notice the faint scent of laundry. Tune in to scents you didn't notice before. What can you smell?

Taste: Examine the piece of fruit. Imagine you're a space alien eating fruit for the first time. Examine it closely. Notice what it looks and smells like. Place it on your tongue: Is it cool, smooth, bumpy? Feel your mouth start to salivate as if that sensation, too, is new. Slowly bite down, noticing the pressure of your teeth on the fruit. Taste it on your tongue, feel the texture in your mouth. Focus all your attention just on your senses. What can you taste?

_____

_____

Check in with your body and emotions:

New stress or anxiety level on a scale from 0 to 10 (0 = none, 5 = moderate, 10 = extreme): _____

New pain rating on a scale from 0 to 10 (0 = none, 5 = moderate, 10 = severe): _____

What did you notice and how did you feel, emotionally and physically?

_____

_____

_____

Schedule a time to practice this week, specifying time and place (*Example: Saturday at 10 a.m. in the park*):

_____

How will you remember to use this tool this week? (*Example: Invite a friend to do it with me*)

_____

Mindful Eating

Do you ever eat in your car, rush through meals, or have no idea how you finished that entire bag of chips while mindlessly watching TV? Most of us eat on autopilot. Some people also *self-soothe* using food, eating to mask or distract themselves from physical and emotional pain. One way to tackle these issues is to try Mindful Eating, which expands upon Five-Senses Mindfulness. Here's how to do it:

HOW TO DO IT

Get a piece of chocolate, keeping it in the wrapper.

Focus all of your attention entirely on this piece of chocolate.

Observe it as if you were an alien from outer space, as if you've never seen anything like this before. Hold it up and inspect it without any judgment.

What colors do you notice? What textures?

_____

Hold it up to your nose and inhale. What does it smell like?

_____

Tune in to your stomach. Notice if you're hungry or full, or if your belly is rumbling. What's your stomach telling you?

_____

Touch the chocolate with your fingertips. Feel the smoothness of the paper or foil. Notice the temperature. Is the foil cool? What does it feel like?

_____

Mindfully unwrap the chocolate. Listen to the sounds the wrapper makes as you open it. What do you hear?

_____

Rub the candy in your fingers and feel the texture. Notice color and shape. Place the chocolate in your mouth without biting or chewing it. Feel it sitting on your tongue. Notice what's happening in your mouth. Are you salivating? Can you taste anything? What's your tongue doing?

_____

Gently bite down on the chocolate. Don't swallow, just feel it in your mouth. Imagine that this is your first time trying chocolate. How would you describe the taste? What's the texture like, is it solid or melting? Notice your teeth and tongue, the saliva at the back of your throat, the urge to swallow. What do you notice?

_____

_____

Chew and swallow. Notice how your lower jaw moves, how your upper jaw stays still, and how your tongue pushes the food to the top of your mouth. How does the texture of the chocolate change? Use all your senses to describe the experience:

_____

_____

Mindful eating can help you slow down and relax, monitor appetite and food intake, and increase pleasure. It can even improve digestion. Did you enjoy the chocolate more when you took the time to appreciate it? (I always do.) You can mindfully eat anytime, anywhere. Try eating an entire meal mindfully and see how it changes your experience of food.

Biofeedback: Hand Warming

As further evidence that your mind affects bodily processes, biofeedback can teach you to heat your hands—just using your mind. Sound like voodoo? It did to me, too…until I learned how to do it! _Biofeedback_ is a scientifically-supported pain-management technique in which we use feedback from our biological systems to bring formerly unconscious processes like heart rate, muscle tension, skin temperature, and pain under conscious control.

We don't normally think of body temperature as something we control: if we're cold, we raise the thermostat or put on a sweater. But not after today! _Hand warming_ is a biofeedback technique in which you use your mind to change your body temperature, teaching your body to alter itself. The science is this: Pain triggers stress, which initiates the fight-or-flight response. This response pulls blood away from extremities (hands and feet) and into your core, to your vital organs. Typically, the more stressed you are, the cooler your extremities—which is why our hands get cold and clammy when we're scared or tense. This also drives the science of lie-detector tests: physiological changes in your hands are picked up by the detector when you get stressed or lie. The more relaxed and safe you feel, the more your blood vessels expand, the more your blood flows to your extremities, and the warmer your hands and feet get.

Relaxation combined with *autogenic phrases* (suggestive statements about physical responses) can turn off the fight-or-flight response, increasing blood flow to your hands. And guess what blood carries? Blood carries heat. Research suggests that biofeedback can reduce various types of chronic pain. In fact, according to the American Migraine Foundation, this technique has been shown to be as effective for migraines and headache as medications, and without the side effects.

HOW TO DO IT

Set aside fifteen minutes for this activity. You can download a recording of this exercise at http://www.newharbinger.com/46448 or have someone read this to you.

For this activity, you'll need a "stress thermometer" to hold between your thumb and index finger to provide feedback about skin temperature. This is different from a fever thermometer. You can get one from Amazon, bio-medical.com, or StressStop.com.

Before starting, hold the thermometer between your thumb and index finger to measure baseline (starting) finger temperature.

Record that here: _____

Now check in with your body and emotions:

Pain rating on a scale from 0 to 10 (0 = none, 5 = moderate, 10 = severe): _____

Stress or anxiety rating on a scale from 0 to 10 (0 = none, 5 = moderate, 10 = extreme): _____

Find a quiet place where you won't be disturbed. Turn off your screens and put them away. Sit somewhere comfortable and quiet, like the couch. Hold the thermometer between your thumb and index finger throughout this exercise. Let your hands hang down by your sides and close your eyes.

Take several slow, deep breaths into your belly. When you inhale, feel your belly rise as it fills with air. Slowly exhale, and feel your body relax.

Remind yourself that you're safe. You have nowhere to go, nothing else to do.

Squeeze your legs, thighs, calves, and ankles together for a count of ten…squeeze harder…then let your body relax.

Next clench your fists and pull them toward your shoulders, squeezing your biceps. Squeeze for a slow count of ten. Let your arms hang loose, and let your body relax.

Bring your attention to the top of your head. Sense into your face—forehead, temples, eyebrows—and let your facial muscles relax. Release your jaw and let it hang open.

Sense into your chest, heart, and lungs. Let your breath be slow. Notice your pulse; feel your heart pumping blood around your body. Allow your heart rate to slow by repeating to yourself: My heart is slow and regular. My heart is slow and regular. *Sense into your neck and shoulders. Let your shoulders drop as if gravity is pulling them down. Let your arms be limp, loose, warm, and relaxed. Repeat to yourself:* My muscles are loose and heavy. My body is heavy and relaxed.

Imagine hollow tubes inside your arms, connecting the tops of your shoulders to the tips of your fingers. Imagine hot, steaming air flowing inside these tubes from the tops of your shoulders, past your elbows, into your forearms, your wrists, the palms of your hands. Feel the hot air filling your hands and pooling in the tips of your fingers. Feel your fingers getting warmer and warmer. Imagine they're getting red and hot. Each time you exhale, imagine hot air flowing down into your hands.

Now imagine hot soup flowing inside your arms. Imagine this steaming hot soup running down your shoulders, past your elbows, into your forearms, the palms of your hands, the tips of your fingers. Feel your fingertips getting hot. Imagine the capillaries and blood vessels in your fingers expanding as your hands get hotter and hotter. Repeat to yourself: My hands are heavy and warm…My hands are heavy and warm. *Let the blood flow into your hands. Feel the heat in your fingertips. Feel your hands throbbing and tingling as they get warmer and warmer.*

Now imagine holding your hands over a campfire. Picture the fire's orange flames, the smell of burning wood. Hold your hands over the fire and feel the heat. As your hands and fingertips get hotter and hotter, feel them tingle and throb. Notice your palms sweating. Feel the flame on your hands until they seem to be red, glowing with heat.

When you're ready, slowly bring your attention back to the room around you. Open your eyes, and look at the thermometer. Look at the insides of your hands and press them to your face. Notice if they're warmer, redder, and sweatier than usual.

Your check-in:

Record your new finger temperature here: _____

Check in with your body and emotions:

New stress or anxiety rating on a scale from 0 to 10 (0 = none, 5 = moderate, 10 = extreme): _____

New pain rating on a scale from 0 to 10 (0 = none, 5 = moderate, 10 = severe): _____

What did you notice and how did you feel? Include any temperature changes.

_____

_____

_____

Behold the power of your mind! If your mind can heat your hands, what could it do to your pain?

_____

_____

Schedule a time to practice tomorrow (*Example: Tomorrow after lunch*):

_____

How will you remember to use this tool this week? (*Example: Set a timer on my phone*)

_____

If you don't notice a significant change the first few times, fear not—like any skill, hand warming takes time and persistence. Try it every day and see how hot your hands get! For more in-depth training, find a local biofeedback provider.

Neurofeedback

A subtype of biofeedback is *neurofeedback* (also called EEG neurofeedback or neurotherapy), in which you get live, real-time feedback about your brain's activity. By applying electrical sensors to your scalp and forehead, neurofeedback providers can read your brain output, called an *EEG*. They can then use this information to help alter stress, anxiety, trauma responses, sleep, and pain. The science is this: neurons, or brain cells, "talk" to each other using electrical energy. This is what thoughts are made of. The brain's electrical activity shows up on EEG monitors as brain waves, translations of the brain's functioning. By getting direct feedback from the brain—for example, determining which areas are particularly active during a specific thought or activity—you can make changes in thoughts and behaviors to change the brain's output.

Imagery

Guided imagery is a mind-body technique that uses mental images to change pain. Imagery allows you to see, smell, hear, feel, and taste things that exist only in your mind—as you do with dreams and memories. Every time you've had a sweaty nightmare, daydreamed in a staff meeting, fantasized about your next vacation, or mentally rehearsed a dance routine, you've used imagery.

Amazingly, research shows that you use the same parts of your brain when *imagining* pain as you do when actually experiencing pain. Mental images trigger physiological responses, so if you remember or imagine a stressful or painful event, your body will initiate a stress response. For example, remembering a medical crisis or vividly imagining a terrifying car crash triggers an emergency response: adrenaline pours into your bloodstream, muscles contract, heart rate increases, pupils dilate, and pain volume increases. Alternatively, if you imagine feeling safe, protected, and calm, and help your body relax, pain volume decreases. In the exercises that follow, you'll use imagery to adjust your pain dial.

Safe-Place Imagery

Have you ever noticed that certain environments, like the dentist's office, can make you feel stressed, while other environments, like a tropical beach, can make you feel relaxed? Well, you don't need to go to the beach to achieve calm: your brain can transport you to peaceful environments just by using imagery. In this exercise, you'll use your five senses to help your mind travel to a safe, relaxing place. This technique teaches your brain that your body is safe, and facilitates mental and physical relaxation to turn the volume down on pain.

HOW TO DO IT

Set aside ten to fifteen minutes for this activity. You can download a recording of this guided imagery exercise at http://www.newharbinger.com/46448 or have someone read it to you.

Check in with your body and emotions:

Pain rating on a scale from 0 to 10 (0 = none, 5 = moderate, 10 = severe): _____

Stress or anxiety level on a scale from 0 to 10 (0 = none, 5 = moderate, 10 = extreme): _____

Find a quiet place to sit or lie down. Turn off your screens and put them away. Close your eyes.

Take a few slow, deep belly breaths. Imagine a safe, relaxing place, preferably in nature, that you've visited or made up. It could be a beach, a wooded trail, a mountain cabin, or even your grandmother's house—as long as it makes you feel safe and relaxed. As you picture this place, use your five senses to complete the imagery exercise below. Use Wendy's example to guide you.

Wendy's Example

My safe, relaxing place is *a warm beach in Mexico.*

Sight: I'm standing on a beautiful stretch of beach in Mexico. As I look around I see colorful beach umbrellas, white seashells, and the ocean stretching before me as far as the eye can see. The water is deep blue and the sand is white. My feet are buried in the warm sand, and waves lap gently at my ankles. Green palm trees with clusters of coconuts line the shore. The sun is setting. The sky is filled with brilliant colors—orange, purple, magenta—as seagulls circle overhead.

Sound: I close my eyes and listen to the sounds of wind and water. I hear boats rocking, kids splashing, waves crashing, people laughing. I hear seagulls calling and palm trees rustling in the warm breeze.

Smell: I inhale the scents of the beach. I smell salt water, seaweed, warm sand, and the faint scent of sunblock on my skin.

Touch: I feel the sun warming my skin and the breeze in my hair. I notice the warm, wet sand between my toes and the cool ocean water lapping against my ankles. I notice the feeling of my clothes on my skin—my wet bathing suit, my dry sundress.

Taste: I taste the saltiness of seawater. I imagine drinking a cold glass of lemonade on this hot day, and feel the cool liquid going down my throat.

Your Example

List three places where you've felt safe and at peace. It can be a place from childhood summers, a relaxing vacation, a fantasyland from a book or movie, or a place you imagine.

1. _____

2. _____

3. _____

Select one of these for this activity.

_____

Sight: Look around your safe place. Describe what it looks like, the time of day, and who's there with you. Notice shapes, colors, and textures. Notice the sky and clouds. Is the sun setting or is it morning? Describe everything you see:

_____

_____

_____

_____

Sound: Use your imagination to tune in to your ears. Describe everything you hear.

_____

_____

_____

Smell: What can you smell?

_____

_____

_____

Touch: What do you feel? Notice textures, temperatures, and sensations.

_____

_____

_____

Taste: What can you taste?

_____

_____

_____

After describing your safe place, let yourself really be there. Completely relax into the scene. If thoughts drift into your head, that's okay—just bring your attention back to the scene. You carry this relaxing place with you wherever you go. You can come back anytime you choose, whether at work or in the doctor's office.

When you've completed this activity, slowly bring your attention back to the room you're in.

Check in with your body and emotions, and notice any changes:

New stress or anxiety level on a scale from 0 to 10 (0 = none, 5 = moderate, 10 = extreme): _____

New pain rating on a scale from 0 to 10 (0 = none, 5 = moderate, 10 = severe): _____

What did you notice as you did this activity?

_____

_____

_____

Schedule a time to practice this week (*Example: After the 10 a.m. staff meeting*):

_____

How will you remember to use guided imagery? (*Example: Tape a note to my mirror*)

_____

This is a helpful activity to use if you have trouble falling asleep. Sleeping is much easier when you feel safe and relaxed. See the list of websites and apps in the "Resources" section for guided audio ideas and sleep meditations.

Self-Healing Imagery

Self-healing imagery uses the power of your imagination to transform pain. Just as your brain can transform environments outside your body using imagery—from a boring bedroom to a Mexican beach—it can also transform the environment inside your body. Have you ever woken up panting and sweaty from a nightmare, your heart pounding? It was just your imagination, but your body reacted with genuine fear as if the threat was real. This happens because of the powerful connection between your imagination (your mind) and your body. Your body responds physiologically to the thoughts and images in your head, resulting in physical changes such as altered heart rate and muscle tension. If you frequently imagine or remember pain, past medical procedures, old traumas, and other stressful events, your nervous system will prepare for an emergency and your pain system will stay on high alert. This turns *up* the pain dial, boosting pain volume. However, taking control of the images in your brain—creating safe, calming images—changes your physiology and turns pain volume *down*.

Try this: Imagine holding a grapefruit. Feel the cool, round shape of the fruit in your palm. Imagine cutting it in half, noticing textures and scents. Squeeze the tart, pink juice into a glass and raise it to your mouth. Inhale the citrus scent. Take a big mouthful of grapefruit juice. Feel the tangy taste and texture on your tongue, the bittersweet juice, the pulp. Imagine the feeling of swallowing. Is your mouth watering as though the experience were real? In response to mental images, your brain's olfactory (smell) and gustatory (taste) centers are activated, triggering the real, physiological response of salivation—even if there's no grapefruit in sight. Try using imagery to alter the activity of your brain's pain centers.

HOW TO DO IT

This imagery technique requires some assistance and creativity. It can be incredibly effective if you're willing to play along. To transform your pain, first read Glenn's, Karen's, and Erik's examples, below, to understand how this technique works. Then fill this out on your own, or ask someone to read the steps to you and ask you the questions listed.

Set aside fifteen minutes for this activity.

Check in with your body and emotions:

Pain rating on a scale from 0 to 10 (0 = none, 5 = moderate, 10 = severe): _____

Stress or anxiety level on a scale from 0 to 10 (0 = none, 5 = moderate, 10 = extreme): _____

Lie down in a quiet place where you won't be interrupted. Turn off your screens and put them away, and close your eyes.

Take a few deep belly breaths. Extend your exhales, breathing out slowly. Belly breathe for a few minutes until your body starts to relax.

Step 1. Travel inside your body now, into the place that hurts, and let yourself focus on the pain. Notice the color, size, shape, and texture of the pain. Notice if it's dark or bright, heavy or light, hot or cool, solid or liquid, static or moving. Try to describe everything you notice about your pain.

Glenn's pain image:

> *Glenn's knee pain is in the shape of a pointy spear tip. It's red, hot, sharp, and prickly. When Glenn closes his eyes and senses into his leg, the pain feels like molten hot liquid, like lava from a*

volcano oozing slowly outward from his knee in concentric circles. This pain is orange, dull, and throbbing.

What does your pain look like? Describe its color, temperature, size, shape, texture, and movement.

_____

_____

_____

This is your *pain image.*

Step 2. Now imagine this part of your body without any pain. When this part of you is healed and pain-free, what does it look like? What color, temperature, size, shape, weight, and texture is it? Is it moving or static? This is your *healing image.*

Glenn's healing image:

> *Without any pain, Glenn imagines that his knee is a smooth, cool, wintry blue. The rest of his leg is cool and pale. It feels solid and there isn't any movement. The circle of sensation in his leg is shrunken and small.*

Your healing image:

_____

_____

_____

Step 3. Imagine you can use magic to transform and heal your pain. What magical process does your body need to transform the pain image into the healing image? Whatever you need to do to change your pain, imagine you can do it! This transformational process can involve a change in color, temperature, size, shape, weight, speed, or texture. You can imagine doing anything to your pain: turn it from orange to blue; cool it or heat it; shrink it or grow it; give it a blast of warm sunlight, icy wind, a deep massage, or a gentle touch; slow it down or speed it up; melt it or harden it; shave off parts or change its shape; change the texture or give it padding.

Glenn's transformational process:

> *To transform his pain from one state to the other, Glenn sends an icy cold waterfall down the inside of his leg. He imagines bathing his fiery knee pain in a cascade of soothing, icy-blue water*

until he can feel the circle of pain healing, shrinking, and cooling. Since his pain image is sharp and pointed, he imagines this powerful, rushing waterfall wearing down the spear until it's smooth.

Your transformational process:

_____

_____

_____

With your eyes still closed, imagine that this self-healing process is actually working. Take a few moments to send this magical healing process to the part of your body that hurts, and picture the pain changing. Imagine that you're transforming your pain.

Slowly bring your attention back to the room.

Check in with your body and emotions:

In what ways did your pain change (color, temperature, size, pain intensity)? How did you feel physically and emotionally?

_____

_____

_____

Check in with your body and emotions:

New stress or anxiety level on a scale from 0 to 10 (0 = none, 5 = moderate, 10 = extreme): _____

New pain rating on a scale from 0 to 10 (0 = none, 5 = moderate, 10 = severe): _____

Schedule a time to practice this week (*Example: Nightly before bed at 11 p.m.*):

_____

How will you remember to use this tool this week? (*Example: Put a note next to my bed*)

_____

Try this imagery technique anew each time you have a pain flare. Pain is always changing! Try not to rely on old pain images or memories to inform your current experience—instead, look inside each time.

Karen's example:

Karen lives with daily migraines. Her pain is a thick, black, oozing fluid that clogs her head between her eyes and makes it throb at the temples. This painful metallic fluid is full of sharp barbs that stab the inside of her skull. When Karen imagines her head healed and pain-free, it's shiny, white, and clear, like an empty glass without any fluid. The texture is smooth and has no barbs. Her head feels light rather than heavy. To transform her pain, Karen vividly imagines two holes magically opening in her temples. These exit holes allow the thick, black fluid to drain out of her head and drip onto the ground. As the heavy metallic fluid flows out, it washes away the sharp barbs at her temples. She imagines that her head feels lighter and that pain lessens as her head becomes weightless, smooth, and clear as glass.

Erik's example:

Erik has irritable bowel syndrome (IBS). It causes chronic pain in his abdomen and intestines below his belly button. He's constantly bloated and gassy, and his stomach is distended. He describes his pain as a dark-green knot in his guts that's tight, twisted, hot, swollen, and lumpy. In his healing image, his stomach and intestines are untangled tubes: long, light pink, relaxed, and healthy. The temperature is cool, and the texture is smooth without any bulges or tangles. To transform the image from painful to pain-free, Erik imagines his intestines relaxing, untangling, loosening, and elongating. He sends his intestines a minty-cool, blue-green breeze to reduce heat and swelling. The cool, wintry tingling of the mint permeates his guts. As this happens, his abdomen gradually changes from dark green to light pink. He imagines the gas bubbles popping and dissolving. As he uses imagery and belly breathes, his stomach relaxes and his pain changes. With everything stretching out, there's more space in his stomach and intestines, and the pain becomes less intense.

Conclusion

Mind-body medicine can change pain. Skills like relaxation, mindfulness, biofeedback, and imagery are powerful tools to control, manage, and cope with pain and symptoms. These techniques exert their effects by changing thoughts, emotions, brain pathways, and physiological systems. In the next chapter, we'll look at how your thoughts can change bodily sensations and pain.

CHAPTER 5

The Biological Connection Between Thoughts and Pain

Have you ever noticed that thoughts like *I'll never get better—nothing will help!* make you feel worse, while telling yourself *It's going to be okay—there's hope!* can make you feel a little bit better? Research shows that stressful, negative thoughts—like the ones we have when we're sick and in pain—can exacerbate and even *cause* health problems and pain. For example, as you learned in chapter 2, negative thoughts and feelings activate stress hormones and neurochemicals that can trigger headaches, stomachaches, and muscle pain; cause lightheadedness and fatigue; exacerbate symptoms; and make you feel worse. Negative thoughts, memories, and emotions also trigger the release of *cytokines*, chemicals that can exaggerate or suppress the body's immune response. This can lead to getting sick, staying sick if you're already ill, and an increase in pain. Last but not least, research shows that negative expectations amplify pain, resulting in increased signaling from the spinal cord to the brain! Negative thoughts aren't just in your head—they also affect your body.

Connecting the Thoughts in Your Head with the Sensations in Your Body

The good news is that there's also a connection between positive thoughts and health. Thoughts and memories that inspire happiness, relaxation, gratitude, self-compassion, optimism, and other positive emotions have been shown to facilitate improved immune functioning, reduced risk of disease, and better overall health. They can also turn down your pain dial, lowering the volume on pain. This means that changing your thoughts can actually change your pain!

There are many ways to harness the power of the mind and transform negative, harmful thoughts into helpful, healing thoughts. These thought-changing CBT techniques are called *cognitive strategies*. In fact, the "C" in CBT stands for *cognitive*, a fancy word for thoughts. Mindfulness practices also emphasize cognitive techniques, such as observing thoughts and focusing attention. Together, these brain- and body-based practices can help you tune in to, identify, and change the negative thoughts associated with pain that keep you feeling miserable, sick, and distressed.

This doesn't mean that pain is "all in your head," that you can "think pain away," or that you can "talk yourself out of" having pain. It also doesn't mean that you should think exclusively cheerful thoughts or never think about your pain. (Have you ever tried to *not* think about a pink elephant? Don't do it! Stop!…good luck.) Pain isn't simply mind-over-matter, and suggesting that it is dismisses its complexity. However, you *can* harness the power of your mind and change your thoughts to change how you feel. In this chapter you'll learn cognitive strategies that can reduce stress and anxiety, lift your mood, shift your attention, and turn down your pain dial. Give them all a try and see which work best for you!

Negative Self-Talk: Pain Voice

We all engage in self-talk—the things we say to ourselves when we think. People with pain and illness often experience *negative self-talk*—pessimistic, catastrophic, critical thoughts about ourselves, life, or pain that bring us down and make us feel worse. We call these negative thoughts *cognitive distortions*, because while they might sound true, they're actually distorted and false. Since negative thoughts impact health and well-being, when we have pain it's particularly important to follow the tenet: "Don't believe everything you think!"

The first step to mastering cognitive distortions is to pay careful attention to your thoughts. If you listen closely, you just might be able to hear what Pain Voice, or Sick Voice, is telling you. *Pain Voice* is your inner bully, the voice in your head that tells you awful, worrisome things about your life and your health. She's pessimistic, catastrophic, critical, and negative. You can recognize Pain Voice because she's very loud! She yells into a megaphone, drowning out all other thoughts—especially the calm, logical, and hopeful ones. The things she tells you sound like the truth, but when you test these thoughts, you discover they're false and distorted. For example, Pain Voice pretends she can predict the future and tells you it's going to be terrible. She says: "You'll never get better. Nothing will ever help you." But since she *can't* actually predict the future (who can?), Pain Voice is a liar.

Pain Voice is also very bossy about what you can and can't do: "You can't go to that football game," or "You can't run, you can't cook, and you definitely can't go out this week." Basically, Pain Voice makes you miserable.

Distorted

Negative

Pain Voice =   *Thoughts*

Critical

Untrue

Picture your Pain Voice and imagine what he or she looks like. Notice that she is not you—she's just a cruel bully in your head who pretends to be in charge. I picture my Pain Voice as a bossy, unattractive blonde with a tight ponytail and lumpy black clothes. She has evil, bulging eyes, dark V-shaped eyebrows, and yells into a megaphone. I call her Beasley. My inner bully, Beasley, is a major *pain*.

She has critical things to say about how I look, how I talk, and the things I say. She enjoys ruminating about catastrophes, pandemics, and natural disasters, vividly imagining every possible worst-case scenario. She constantly comments on my pain and health, and gets particularly loud before procedures and doctor's appointments. She always predicts these will go terribly and be unbearably painful. She constantly tries to trap me with her negativity.

Picture your Pain Voice and describe what he or she looks like. Pain Voice can be male or female, old or young, tall or short.

_____

_____

Name your Pain Voice.

_____

In what situations do you hear him or her the most?

1. _____

2. _____

3. _____

Example: John's Pain Voice

John's kidney stones usually rank 7 out of 10 on the pain scale and typically pass after a few weeks. However, during a recent flare, pain persisted for three months. John heard the thought: Something's wrong; this pain is from something else! What if it's prostate cancer? His pain immediately shot to 10 out of 10, becoming so intense that he doubled over. His wife rushed him to the ER, where the doctor conducted an imaging test. As soon as John saw the stone on the screen and got medical confirmation that this was the likely source of his discomfort, his pain immediately dropped to a 3. Said John: "My catastrophic thoughts and fears about what was happening to my body were neutralized when I saw the stone, and this instantly changed my pain."

Name a time your thoughts affected your pain:

_____

_____

_____

Tune in to your Pain Voice and really listen hard. You've heard her a million times before. What kinds of negative, catastrophic, self-defeating things does she say to you? Here are some common Pain Voice thoughts. Circle the ones that are familiar, and add your own:

I'm broken.

My life is always going to be like this.

Nothing will ever help me.

There's no point trying this treatment because nothing else has helped.

I can't do anything on days I'm sick or in pain.

This pain is a punishment for _____.

Pain is my fault: I deserve this.

I'm worthless.

I'm not good enough. I'm not doing enough.

Nobody understands what I'm going through.

My body hates me. My body is my enemy.

I'll never get better.

Pain is an indication that my body is broken.

If I (exercise, weed, go sailing), I'll reinjure myself.

My friends have all moved on without me.

I'm a burden to my friends and family.

My life sucks.

I'm so far behind at work that I'll never catch up.

People think I'm faking.

Pain is ruining my life.

Pain is ruining my future.

Bad things always happen to me.

I'll never be in shape like I was before.

Tomorrow (next week, next year) is going to be as bad as today.

The only thing that can help is medication.

I can't live with this pain.

_____

_____

_____

_____

Extreme Negative Thoughts: Suicidality

It's common to have negative thoughts when living with chronic pain. Indeed, sadness, stress, and anxiety are normal responses to an abnormal situation: the body wasn't built to experience daily, ongoing pain for months and years on end. But sometimes the stress and sadness can become too much to bear. Risk of suicidality is significantly higher in the chronic-pain population. If you have thoughts about ending your life or feel like you can't go on, now is the time to get the support and help you deserve. Medical interventions alone are not enough to get well—you must also take care of your thoughts and emotions. Call a suicide hotline like the National Suicide Prevention Hotline (1-800-273-8255 as of this publication), text "HOME" to 741741 on your cell phone (Crisis Text Line; also try the website www.crisistextline.org), or go to a local hospital. Call a friend or doctor and ask for help. Hire a therapist. Try a live or online therapy group for depression, anxiety, addiction, or chronic pain. There's no shame in taking good care of yourself in this moment of need—in fact, it's the most courageous thing you can do.

The Voice of Wellness: Wise Voice

Fear not, brave friend—because all hope is not lost. You have another voice inside you: your *Wise Voice*. She is strong, logical, calm, and gentle, and helps you feel *better* instead of worse. If you tune in, you can recognize her encouraging, compassionate, and kind messages. As someone who genuinely loves you, she sounds like a family member, partner, or close friend. Since Wise Voice is quiet and soft-spoken, your loud, obnoxious Pain Voice usually drowns her out.

$$
\textit{Wise Voice} = \begin{array}{c} \textit{Logical} \\ \textit{Balanced} \\ \textit{Compassionate} \\ \textit{True} \end{array} \textit{Thoughts}
$$

Picture your Wise Voice and bring her to life. She lives inside of you and is always with you. My Wise Voice is an older woman with silver hair woven into a bun. She has a broad, sturdy back and her arms are muscular and strong. She sits tall with legs crossed, peacefully smiling, eyes closed. She is wise, calm, and confident. I call her Clara because she's clear and bright. She speaks calmly and quietly—but I can hear her when I tune in. She tends to show up most when I'm giving friends advice or counseling children. She's the loving voice of comfort, kindness, and wisdom I access when speaking with people I love.

Picture your Wise Voice. What does he or she look like? Wise Voice can be male or female, old or young, tall or short.

_____

_____

Name your Wise Voice.

_____

In what situations do you hear him or her the most?

1. _____

2. _____

3. _____

To regain strength and heal, we need to quiet Pain Voice and replace her with Wise Voice. But how?

Prove Pain Voice Wrong in Three Steps

To mute Pain Voice and shut her down, you must first catch her (Beasley, is that you?) and thoughtfully determine, or check, whether or not what she's saying is true. What if the thought isn't a fact? What if the only purpose of the thought is to hurt you, weaken you, and fill you with fear and self-doubt?

Because negative thoughts increase pain, it's critical to make sure that you don't thoughtlessly, automatically believe them. As soon as you recognize Pain Voice (*It IS you, you beastly bully!*), you gain the power to change negative thoughts into more helpful, healing, Clara-clear, Wise Voice thoughts.

Here's an overview of the three steps to shift from Pain Voice to Wise Voice. We'll use the rest of this chapter to become experts in steps 1 and 2. You'll learn how to change thoughts (step 3) in chapter 6.

- **Step 1: Catch it.** Get familiar with your recurring Pain Voice thoughts so you can *recognize* and catch them the instant they happen. Slow them down so they're no longer automatic. Remember your biopsychosocial *triggers* from chapter 1—what situations, behaviors, feelings, and events activate negative thoughts?

- **Step 2: Check it.** Once you've caught Pain Voice, *question her* to determine whether that negative thought is true. Check to see whether it's distorted, and gather logical evidence against it. Then challenge thoughts that are harmful, exaggerated, or flat-out untrue.

- **Step 3: Change it.** Use the evidence you gather to *replace* Pain Voice with the voice of wellness, your Wise Voice. At first you may not hear Wise Voice very often, but she's even more powerful than Pain Voice. Once you start attending to her kind, rational, compassionate messages, she'll get even stronger.

Step 1: Catch Pain Voice Using Thinking Traps

It's normal to have a loud, negative Pain Voice when you're sick or in pain. These thoughts sound like the truth (*My life sucks!*) and trap you into believing them, but they're actually stressful, exaggerated, and untrue. Pain Voice thoughts are therefore called *cognitive distortions*, or *thinking traps*. Thinking traps are the La Brea Tar Pits of your mind. The La Brea Tar Pits are pits of natural asphalt in Los Angeles, California. They bubbled up to the surface from deep within the earth during the last Ice Age, burning hot and lethally sticky, trapping living animals, pulling them below the surface, and suffocating them. Similarly, cognitive distortions are sticky, dangerous traps that try to pull you down and smother you with pain and negativity. *Don't let them.* Thinking traps make you feel depressed, spike stress and anxiety, wreck self-esteem, turn up the pain dial, and trap you in unhealthy coping behaviors such as avoiding people, exercise, hobbies, and work. Thinking traps are dangerous because they *feel* true even if they're not *factually* true.

So how do you pull your mind out of the tar, stop these distorted thoughts, and distinguish traps from truth? Answer: You become a "thought detective," capturing thoughts and examining evidence. One way to recognize a trap is to notice how the thought makes you feel. Is the thought *helpful,* or is it *harmful?* Check the list of Pain Voice thoughts you circled earlier—do they make you feel hopeful and inspired, or discouraged and miserable? You can recognize these traps because they make you feel worried, sad, hopeless, or angry. Go through the following thinking traps and identify familiar ones. See if you can tease out why they're harmful and how they make you feel.

Black-or-White Thoughts. This is a type of extreme thinking in which things seem black or white, right or wrong, wonderful or terrible, all or nothing. There's no middle ground. If something isn't perfect or doesn't go as planned, you see it as a total failure. For example: *That treatment didn't work; therefore, I can't be helped. I can be happy only if I don't have pain. I'm right, so anyone who disagrees with me is wrong.*

Do thoughts like these sound familiar?   Y   N

Name one of your black-or-white thoughts:

_____

Is this thought **helpful** or **harmful**? (Circle one.)

How does it make you feel?

_____

This thought is a trap because the world doesn't exist in extremes. It's rare that you're at one extreme or the other, either 100% right (black) or 100% wrong (white). It's equally as rare for pain to *always* be a 10 out of 10 (black) or to always be a 0 out of 10 (white). Most of the time, you're somewhere in the middle (gray!). When you notice yourself going "black or white," remind yourself to "go gray" and imagine possibilities in the middle.

Overgeneralization. This is a form of black-or-white thinking in which you believe that a single negative event, like a pain flare or a hard day, is an enduring, lifelong pattern. You use words like "always/never," "everybody/nobody," "best/worst," and "all/nothing." For example: *I can never do anything when I'm sick or in pain. I can't work. Nobody will ever hire me. My (whole) life sucks!* Or you may use this as a weapon of self-judgment: *If I don't clean the house today, I'm a terrible parent.*

Do thoughts like these sound familiar?   **Y   N**

Name one of your overgeneralizations:

_____

Is this thought **helpful** or **harmful**? (Circle one.)

How does it make you feel?

_____

This thought is a trap because one negative event isn't representative of all events. Does *everything* about your life suck because you had one bad day, or even a bad week? Is it true that *nobody* will *ever* hire you? I call these *warning words* because they're dangerous exaggerations and rarely true, and indicate that you've fallen into a sticky thinking trap. Replace black-or-white warning words with balanced words like "some," "sometimes," or even "a few." For example: *This was a tough week, but not everything was bad. Some good things happened, too.*

Filtering. You focus on negative information and events and ignore the positive. You accept criticism and negativity from others while rejecting compliments and kindnesses. For example, you get many positive comments on a presentation, but one person is critical and says it was terrible. You obsess about this negative comment for days and ignore the positive feedback.

Do thoughts like these sound familiar?   **Y   N**

Name a time you filtered:

_____

Is this thought **helpful** or **harmful**? (Circle one.)

How does it make you feel?

This thought is a trap because your brain selectively (and erroneously) focuses on negative information and ignores the good. Why does one bad comment count more than a good one? You may dismiss a compliment by thinking, *He's just being nice because he's my friend*, but what if he means it? It's easy to accept criticism over compliments, but if you accept only negative information, your mood and self-esteem will crash.

Misinterpretation. You misinterpret and catastrophize body signals and symptoms, believing they're indicators of more serious conditions. Common examples include interpreting symptoms of anxiety, like chest pain or racing heart, as a sign you're having a heart attack; interpreting stress-based stomachaches as an illness; or deciding that tingling in your arms or legs means you're having a stroke rather than an anxiety attack. You might also believe that all pain indicates that your condition is worsening or that your body is at war with you. For example: *My body hates me.* Or, *This headache is a sign of a brain tumor.* On an airplane, you might think, *This leg pain is due to a blood clot!*

Do thoughts like these sound familiar? Y N

When have you misinterpreted body signals?

Is this thought **helpful** or **harmful**? (Circle one.)

How does it make you feel?

This thought is a trap because misinterpreting body signals leads to anxious, catastrophic thoughts that amplify pain. (See "Catastrophizing," below.) Before you jump to conclusions, try listing likely alternatives. Is it more likely you're having a heart attack, or that you're anxious? Remember, emotions aren't just in your head—they also come out in your body. Everyday stress, like the stress of living with chronic pain, can cause muscle tension and vasoconstriction (reduced blood flow), leading to headaches and body aches. And that stomachache may be better explained by your *enteric nervous system*, the gut–brain system that serves as an emotion center. Maybe that leg pain you feel on the airplane is due to sitting for six hours, not a blood clot! Not all physical sensations indicate something medically dangerous.

Mind Reading. You believe people are thinking negative things about you without even asking them. You "know" what's in other people's minds even though you have no evidence. For example: *She doesn't like me.* Or, *Everyone thinks I'm faking.*

Do thoughts like these sound familiar?   **Y   N**

When have you read minds?

_____

Is this thought **helpful** or **harmful**? (Circle one.)

How does it make you feel?

_____

This thought is a trap because while it would be amazing to read minds, chances are you don't have that superpower (sorry!). Want to test it out? Ask someone to think of a number between zero and one hundred and try to guess it on the first try. If you can't do it, this means you *can't actually read minds.* The only way to know what other people are thinking is to ask. Assuming other people are thinking bad things about you is a surefire way to feel anxious, angry, and upset.

Fortune-telling. You believe you can see into the future and predict that things are going to go badly. Before a procedure you think, *This is going to go terribly.* If you're sick or in pain, you think, *Nothing can help me. This treatment won't work.* Or, *My future is full of pain.*

Do thoughts like these sound familiar?   **Y   N**

When have you tried to predict the future?

_____

Is this thought **helpful** or **harmful**? (Circle one.)

How does it make you feel?

_____

This thought is a trap because…*Wait!* You can predict the future? Wow, we're gonna be rich! Quick, what are next week's winning lottery numbers?…What? You don't know? (Sigh.) Well, I guess that means you can't predict the future. If you're sick or in pain, predicting a negative, pain-filled future will only make you feel anxious, depressed, and hopeless. (If you *can* predict the future, please call me.)

Permanence. This is a type of fortune-telling in which you believe things are permanent, and that the way things are right now is the way they'll always be—forever. For example: *My pain will never go away.* Or, *I'll never get better.*

Do thoughts like these sound familiar?   **Y**   **N**

What thoughts of permanence have you had?

_____

Are these thoughts **helpful** or **harmful**? (Circle one.)

How do they make you feel?

_____

These thoughts are a trap because humans are great at believing that now = forever! The only thing certain about life is that things constantly change. Pain changes all the time, so why couldn't it change for the better? Even if pain continues, are you positive you can't improve the way you manage it? Believing that pain and suffering are permanent and beyond your capacity to tolerate can lead to depression, anxiety, hopelessness, and even suicidality. Remember: you can't predict the future!

Catastrophizing. This is when Pain Voice magnifies or exaggerates the threat or seriousness of pain and symptoms, leading to feelings of helplessness and hopelessness. These thoughts may repeat incessantly, leading you to believe that the worst thing that *can* happen is *going to* happen. For example, you wake up with pain and think, *This unbearable pain is never going to end. It's ruining my life.* Or, *I've had pain all month, which means I'm getting worse!* Or, *I can't stand this! A life with pain just isn't worth living.*

Do thoughts like these sound familiar?   **Y**   **N**

Name two of your catastrophic thoughts.

1. _____

2. _____

Are these thoughts **helpful** or **harmful**? (Circle one.)

How do they make you feel?

_____

Catastrophic thoughts are dangerous because they trigger stress and fear. Probability science tells us that the worst possible outcome isn't actually the most likely outcome—if anything, it's highly *unlikely*. Catastrophic thoughts can show up as rumination (constantly thinking the same thoughts over and over again), magnification (magnifying the threat that something very serious will happen, or predicting the *worst possible version* of the future), and helplessness. Research shows that catastrophizing not only contributes to heightened levels of pain and emotional distress, it also increases the probability that pain will persist over an extended period of time. When you catastrophize, you're more likely to avoid activity, withdraw, and hole up—which only make pain worse.

Hurt = Harm. This is believing that all pain accurately reflects tissue damage, even in the absence of concrete evidence of bodily harm: believing that pain is your body's way of telling you that it's damaged even when it isn't. For example: *When I move my back it hurts; therefore, moving must be bad.* Or, *Going for a walk with a headache is bad for me.* Or, *My body is in danger, so I must protect it by staying home.*

Do thoughts like these sound familiar?   **Y   N**

When have you assumed that hurt = harm?

_____

Is this thought **helpful** or **harmful**? (Circle one.)

How does it make you feel?

_____

This thought is a trap because *hurt* and *harm* are not the same. It's easy to believe that pain is an accurate indicator of tissue damage, but it isn't. Sometimes the brain makes pain to protect you when no protection is actually required. Of course, there are times when pain—particularly acute, short-term pain—indicates bodily harm and requires immediate action. But chronic pain is often a false alarm created by an overly alert and hypersensitive pain system. In fact, movement and exercise are critically important components of chronic-pain treatment! Activity and stimulation desensitize brain and body, and help you conquer pain.

Labeling. This is when you call yourself a negative name or give yourself a label. For example, instead of saying *I made a mistake*, you think to yourself, *I'm an idiot*. You may call yourself ugly, stupid, or fat. If you haven't been able to do much lately, you may think, *I'm lazy*. People with pain or illness sometimes think, *I'm broken*.

Do thoughts like these sound familiar?   Y   N

Write two names, or labels, you've called yourself recently:

_____

Are these thoughts **helpful** or **harmful**? (Circle one.)

How do they make you feel?

_____

These thoughts are a trap because calling yourself names only makes you feel bad about yourself. When self-esteem crashes, mood worsens, anxiety spikes, and pain volume intensifies. Be loving and kind to yourself instead…being sick and in pain is hard enough as it is!

Biomedical Bias. This means seeking exclusively biomedical explanations and treatments while neglecting cognitive, emotional, social, and contextual factors; believing that your pain requires a constant, unremitting search for answers and diagnoses from physicians even after years of tests and procedures. For example: *I won't get better until I have a medical explanation for the cause of my pain*. Or, *The doctors are just missing it. I know my back is injured*. Or, *The only possible solutions for my pain are pills and procedures*.

Do thoughts like these sound familiar?   Y   N

What biomedical biases do you have?

1. _____

2. _____

Are these beliefs **helpful** or **harmful**? (Circle one.)

How do they make you feel?

_____

It's important to seek biomedical solutions for pain and illness, and hopefully you've found some great providers and tools that have helped. However, these thoughts are a trap because *pain isn't purely biomedical.* Instead, chronic pain is biopsychosocial, the product of biological, psychological, and social factors that create and maintain a cycle of suffering. Continuously seeking exclusively biomedical explanations and treatments keeps you stuck in a cycle of anxiety and disappointment when pain doesn't resolve. Chronic pain isn't just in the body; it's also in the *brain.* Effectively treating chronic pain requires addressing all parts of this biopsychosocial issue, including thoughts, emotions, and coping behaviors.

Powerlessness. You believe that things just happen *to* you and that you have no control over life or events. You believe that your pain is controlled exclusively by external forces, that you are utterly powerless over it, and that the only solutions for it exist outside of you. For example: *I have no control over my pain. Pain decides what I do and don't do.* Or, *I can manage my pain only if I take something for it.* Or, *My doctors are the only ones who can help me.*

Do thoughts like these sound familiar?   **Y   N**

What thoughts of powerlessness have you had?

_____

Are these thoughts **helpful** or **harmful**? (Circle one.)

How do they make you feel?

_____

These thoughts are Pain Voice's way of stealing control. As long as you feel helpless and powerless, pain gets to be in charge! Research shows that having an "external locus of control"—believing that pain and other events are controlled by external forces (such as providers, luck, destiny)—is associated with poorer health outcomes, less treatment success, high stress, and higher pain, while having an "internal locus of control," or a belief in your own power and self-efficacy, is actually associated with better health, better treatment efficacy, lower anxiety, less pain, and less disability. If you feel powerless, you're more likely to give up. If you believe in your own power, you'll marshal your inner strength and use your skills (like the ones in this book!) to change your pain.

Emotional Reasoning. This is when you confuse thoughts and emotions for facts. For example: *I'm anxious and worried—something bad must be happening.* Or, *I feel hopeless; therefore, things are hopeless.*

Do thoughts like these sound familiar?   **Y   N**

When have you used emotional reasoning?

_____

Is this thought **helpful** or **harmful**? (Circle one.)

How does it make you feel?

_____

Your emotions are real and valid. However, emotions and thoughts are not facts. You may legitimately feel hopeless and subsequently have thoughts of hopelessness, but *this doesn't mean that all hope is actually lost.* It's important not to confuse emotions for facts. In fact, there is zero evidence that your pain, or your life, is hopeless.

Step 2. Check Pain Voice Using Detective Questions

Once you've caught a negative thought, how do you determine whether it's a trap or the truth? Answer: you question, or *check*, Pain Voice. If you continue to accept these thoughts as facts, pain volume will stay high. Instead, assess their truthfulness using the following Detective Questions. These logical, fact-based questions help you access your Wise Voice—the kind, calm voice that knows the truth. The moment you recognize that a thought is a thinking trap, you gain the power to change it. Here's how Cristian applied Detective Questions to catch and check his Pain Voice:

Cristian's Story

After an accident kept Cristian out of work most of the year, he worried about losing his job. As he missed more work, his boss became more displeased, and Cristian grew increasingly concerned. He felt overwhelmed and started having anxiety attacks. Then Cristian started CBT and learned cognitive strategies to help manage pain and anxiety. After writing down his Pain Voice thoughts, he began recognizing them in his head. His Pain Voice was an abusive, beer-swilling thug he called Paul. Paul the Pain Voice dressed in a dirty, beer-stained T-shirt, smelled foul, and constantly criticized Cristian. Paul sounded a lot like Cristian's dad. Cristian noticed that sometimes he believed, and got trapped by, these negative thoughts. The thought that trapped him most was, I missed so much work that I'm going to get fired, never work again, and have to live on the streets. *This thought sounded true, even though it was harmful and made him feel terrible. Because Cristian caught this fortune-telling prediction, he was able to recognize and check Paul the Pain Voice, who was trying to keep him anxious and miserable.*

Cristian used the following **Detective Questions** to determine whether this prediction was the truth or a trap.

Thought: I missed so much work that I'm going to get fired, never work again, and have to live on the streets.

Detective Questions:

Is it a fact? (Note: A fact means it is unquestionably, absolutely, certainly true.)

No, it isn't a fact that I'm going to lose my job and be homeless.

Are you predicting bad things?

Yes, this is a prediction. Since I can't predict the future, this fortune-telling thought is a trap.

Are you using a warning word (all/nothing, everyone/no one, always/never/forever, best/worst)?

"Never" is a warning word. This thought is a trap.

What evidence do you have that this might *not* be true?

My brother lost his job last year and he isn't homeless. People lose jobs all the time and they find new ones, including people living with pain.

What has happened in the past?

I've been fired from at least four jobs in my life and I'm still not out on the streets.

What's the likelihood this bad thing will actually happen? (Try to give a percentage; for example, 1% = 1/100.)

The percent chance that I'm going to be homeless and never work again is probably zero. If I applied to a hundred jobs, including some I'm overqualified for, I'd certainly land one of them.

What else—neutral or positive—might happen in this situation other than what you're predicting?

Neutral: Maybe nothing would happen. I might not get fired. Or, if I do, I could find a similar job with similar pay, and just keep living my life without any major changes.

Positive: This could be a blessing in disguise. I don't like this job anyway. I could find a better one with better pay and a better boss.

What's the worst-case scenario? Could you handle it?

Worst-case scenario would be losing this job and not being able to find another one for a long time. That would suck but it wouldn't destroy me. I'd survive. I'd ask my sister for help, search online for resources, email my contact list for leads, and wouldn't give up. So yes—I could handle it.

What would you say to a close friend or a family member who expressed this concern to you?

I'd say: "Your accident and its aftermath have been terrible. Pain has interfered with your life in a very real way. It makes sense you're worried about losing your job and becoming destitute. Those are legitimate fears. I know it's been hard going from a good job to barely working. But this injury hasn't changed who you are: you're still smart, competent, and capable. If you want to get another job, you will. You've done it before, and you can do it again. You have a support system and you're not alone. Your worry is reasonable, but it's not factual. Don't let Paul the Pain Voice get you down!"

Now it's your turn. Pick a thinking trap or Pain Voice thought and write it in the space below. Challenge this thought using the Detective Questions. Determine why this thought is flawed, and see if you can prove why it's a trap and not the truth.

Your negative thought: _____

_____

Detective Questions:

Is it a fact? (Note: a fact means it is unquestionably, absolutely, certainly true.)

_____

Are you predicting bad things?

_____

Are you using a warning word (all/nothing, everyone/no one, always/never/forever, best/worst)?

What evidence do you have that this thought might *not* be true?

What has happened in the past?

What's the likelihood that this bad thing will actually happen? Try to give a percentage. (Reminder: 1% = 1/100. What this means is that out of every hundred instances, the terrible consequence you're predicting happens once. For example, if you predict there's a 1% chance that your airplane will crash, this means that out of every hundred planes that take off globally each day, one crashes.)

What else—neutral or positive—might happen in this situation other than what you're predicting?

What's the worst-case scenario? Could you handle it?

_____

_____

_____

What would you say to a close friend or a family member who expressed this concern to you?

_____

_____

_____

Conclusion

Pain wants your power. One of the ways it tries to take it is by dominating your thoughts and commandeering your mind. _Don't let it._ Because negative, catastrophic, and distorted thoughts turn up the pain dial, it's important for you to take control of self-talk. When you learn to recognize Pain Voice and start challenging her, you begin to take your power back. The next step is to strengthen and empower your inner Wise Voice—the calm, centered, logical part of you that fights back against pain, helping you feel better instead of worse. But how? In the next chapter, you'll learn Step 3: transforming your thought to transform your pain.

CHAPTER 6

Cognitive Strategies: Pain and Your Brain

In the last chapter you learned the many ways that thoughts affect pain. You uncovered the harmful, distorted thoughts generated by Pain Voice that keep you feeling stuck, hopeless, and defeated. You caught Pain Voice (Step 1) and learned to check, challenge, and prove her wrong using Detective Questions (Step 2). The next step, Step 3, is to use cognitive strategies to *change* Pain Voice into another voice entirely. This chapter will teach you to tune in to your inner Wise Voice; to create factual, helpful responses to Pain Voice; and to use coping thoughts to protect yourself and fight back. You'll also learn to use self-compassion as a tool for wellness. These strategies can change your brain to change your pain!

Step 3: Change Pain Voice

Turning down the pain dial means having power over what you think and when, determining which thoughts you embrace and which you discard. Use the cognitive techniques in this chapter to transform thoughts, emotions, coping abilities, and physical sensations as you navigate the road to health.

Thought Tracking

To counteract Pain Voice, start tracking your thoughts. First, list your negative, critical thoughts every time you hear one. Note whether these thoughts are helpful or harmful, whether they're the truth or a trap. Next, write out the answers to the Detective Questions—these are your Wise Voice responses. Wise Voice responses should include evidence indicating *why* Pain Voice is wrong. At the end of this activity, you'll have a Wise Voice response ready for combat—so that every time you hear Pain Voice from now on, you'll be prepared to retaliate. Your Wise Voice grows stronger every time you use it, and Pain Voice grows weaker every time you explode it.

Pain Voice Log

Situation	Pain Voice	Helpful or Harmful?	Trap or Truth	Wise Voice
Resuming work after a month out	My boss is angry about my absences and will critique everything I do. I'm going to get stressed out, my back will spasm, and I'll have to go home. This is going to be awful.	Harmful	Trap	I can't predict the future or read minds. My boss won't critique everything I do— he may have an attitude, but I can handle that. I've handled his attitude for 3 years and I've handled worse! Returning to work might not be all bad. If I'm in pain, I know what to do: I'll take a break, use a heating pad, stretch, and distract.
Pain flare-up	I can't handle this!	Harmful	Trap	This negative prediction is not a fact. I've had 80 flare-ups this year alone, and I handled all of them. I've proven that I'm strong and resilient. There is a 0% chance I can't handle this.

Pain Voice Log

Situation	Pain Voice	Helpful or Harmful?	Trap or Truth	Wise Voice

Go Gray

Pain Voice and Sick Voice love speaking in black-or-white thinking traps. For example, it's easy to think that having pain or being sick means you can do *nothing*, while being pain-free means you can do *everything*. These exaggerated, extreme thoughts limit your ability to manage pain and live your life.

One method for tackling these tricky, sticky thoughts is to consider: What happens when you mix black (nothing) and white (everything) together? You get *gray*. Indeed, the majority of life is lived between black and white, in various shades of gray. When you notice yourself thinking in extremes, try to "go gray" and imagine possibilities in the middle. If extremely high-pain days mean zero activity and extremely low-pain days mean lots of activity, what options exist in the middle on days with *some* pain?

Here's an example:

Black Thought
When I have pain, I can't do *anything*.
No work, stay home.
Stop playing cello.
No hiking.
Don't see any friends.

White Thought
When I'm pain-free, I can do *everything*.
Work 9-5 daily.
Play cello every evening for 2 hours.
Hike 5 miles every weekend.
See friends regularly.

Gray Thought
On a day with *some* pain, I can do *some* things.
Work for half day.
Play cello for 10 minutes Mon, Wed, Fri.
Hike for 15 minutes Saturday morning.
Invite one friend over this weekend to watch a zombie movie.

Marjorie's Gray Thought

Marjorie was a dancer. She'd been dancing since she was a child, belonged to a dance team, and regularly competed in regional competitions. However, she'd stopped dancing when she was diagnosed with a neuromuscular disease that impacted coordination, balance, and physical strength. It also caused episodes of severe pain, particularly in her legs. After months of treatment with medication and physical therapy, her balance and coordination improved enough that her doctors cleared her to gradually start dancing again. But Marjorie was scared that her symptoms would worsen if she was active, and believed she needed to keep resting. She hadn't gone to practice or seen her dance team since her diagnosis because it was too hard to watch them compete without her. On bad days she curled up on the couch with her cats and watched hours of TV. She was miserable. The longer this went on, the less energy and motivation she had.

When Marjorie learned about "going gray," she realized that Pain Voice was saying that she'd never dance again and that she should quit. Her black-or-white thought was, "When I'm symptomatic I can't dance at all, but when I'm symptom-free I can dance daily." She developed a plan to try dancing for ten minutes on days with some symptoms.

On Monday she woke with fatigue, pain, and fear. She considered skipping dance as usual, but reminded herself that "a day with some symptoms means I can do some things." She put on her dance clothes and did ten minutes of warm-up exercises, holding on to a bar for support. She was out of shape and had some pain, but it felt good to put on dance shoes, great to stretch and move her body, and miraculous to discover that she didn't need to give up her love of dancing just because she had neuromuscular disease. She felt so encouraged that she decided to dance again the next day.

Practice going gray using the following table. Enter your black and white thoughts and corresponding activity levels. Then consider: How can you go gray on days with some symptoms? Think of different categories like work, hobbies, social life, exercise, and activities of daily living (such as laundry, cooking, or mowing). Consider all shades of gray: you might have a medium-to-high pain day (dark gray) that allows for a little less activity, and a low-to-medium pain day (light gray) that allows for a little more activity. Use units of time and other measurements to make activity goals specific, realistic, and achievable. For example, a low-to-medium pain goal might be to dance for fifteen minutes four days this week at 6 p.m.

Go Gray

Black	Dark Gray	Light Gray	White
If pain is high, I can't do anything.	*If pain is medium-high, I can do some things.*	*If pain is low-medium, I can do some things.*	*If I don't have any pain, I can do everything.*
If pain is high this week, I can't dance at all.	If pain is medium-high, I'll dance for 5 minutes three days this week (M, W, F) at 6 p.m.	If pain is low-medium, I'll dance for 15 minutes four days this week (M, W, F, Sun) at 6 p.m.	If I have no pain this week, I'll dance every day after work for 30 minutes.

What Ifs

We all know the What Ifs: *What if things go terribly wrong? What if this procedure fails? What if I can never walk again? What if my pain gets worse?* As you've probably guessed, "What If" thoughts belong to your anxious, catastrophic Pain Voice. One way to squash these is to "What If" the opposite. That is: assert the same What If, but generate an opposite outcome—even if it sounds untrue. Remember, if a terribly negative outcome is possible—which is what Pain Voice wants you to believe—a positive outcome is possible, too.

Example: What if this goes badly?

Opposite: What if this goes better than I ever imagined?

Example: What if I try to walk and I fall?

Opposite: What if I try to walk and succeed, proving to myself—and the world—that I can do it?

Note that you aren't *predicting* a positive outcome or assuming that things will be grand; you're simply questioning whether a positive opposite is possible, and envisioning what it might look like. This practice gives your brain a chance to imagine this outcome as a reality. Imagining and mentally rehearsing an outcome can actually change neural pathways, increase motivation and intention, and make that outcome more likely to occur. Defeating negative "What Ifs" can also lift your mood and inspire hope. Try it here, noting how each thought makes you feel.

What If Tracking

What If Thought	How does this thought make you feel?	What If Opposite	How does this thought make you feel?
What if this treatment program fails?	Anxious, overwhelmed, discouraged.	What if it goes well and helps me feel better?	Optimistic, hopeful, motivated.

Coping Thoughts

Just as negative thoughts discourage you and make symptoms feel worse, *coping thoughts* can help you feel better. Coping thoughts are soothing, encouraging, and calming statements that help you get through your day, accomplish goals, and manage pain so that you can function. They come from your kind, helpful Wise Voice, and notify your brain that your body is safe. Coping thoughts help break the stress-pain cycle, turn off the fight-or-flight response, and turn the volume down on pain.

Coping thoughts are useful when Pain Voice gets loud, like when you have a doctor's appointment, a deadline, or a pain flare. As soon as you feel stressed, anxious, or angry and start hearing negative, unhelpful thoughts—pause, take a breath, and tell Pain Voice to STOP! Picture a red stop sign or flashing red light. Then use a coping thought instead. Coping thoughts sound like this:

I've had hundreds of pain flares and bad days in my life, and I survived *all of them*. I'll survive this one, too.

I'm in charge of my body and mind. I can help myself heal.

I'll distract myself with (a TV show, a game, my dog, a friend) for twenty minutes and see if it helps.

I know how to cope with this.

All sensations are temporary. This too shall pass!

It's going to be okay. I'm going to be okay.

I can use my self-soothing plan and other workbook techniques to lower pain volume.

I'm not alone. I have friends, family, community, and online support groups to help me get through this.

I'm doing the best I can. I'm working on getting better every day.

I'm strong. I can get through this.

Just breathe.

What are five soothing, reassuring things you can say to yourself when you're anxious, hurting, or hearing Pain Voice? You can use the coping thoughts above, make up your own, or imagine the sweet, comforting things you'd say to beloved friends or family members.

1. _____

2. _____

3. _____

4. _____

5. _____

Put a copy of your coping thoughts on your bathroom mirror, your bedroom wall, and your fridge. Practice them daily so they become as familiar as your worried thoughts. Just as your Pain Voice got strong with a lot of use, your inner Wise Voice needs a chance to strengthen, too. The more you use her, the stronger she'll get—until she's loud enough to drown out Pain Voice!

Heal Using Self-Compassion

Compassion is the act of being loving, kind, and empathic. *Self-compassion* is directing this loving empathy toward yourself. It may sound simple, but it can be very hard to do—especially for those of us with loud inner bullies, critics, or Pain Voices (*I'm talking to you, beastly Beasley*). One trick for practicing self-compassion is to think of the kindest, most compassionate person in your life and invite her into your head.

Who's the kindest, most thoughtful, most compassionate person in your life? Mine is my childhood friend Amanda. Amanda always has the most kind, supportive, loving things to say no matter what the situation. She forgives my mistakes and embraces my imperfections. She's miraculously able to tap into feelings of empathy and concern even when she herself is stressed. Amanda has come to embody my inner *Compassionate Voice*—the loving, sweet voice in my head that encourages me and lifts me up when I'm feeling sick, sad, or unmotivated—or when I feel the urge to criticize and abuse myself.

Research shows that practicing self-compassion can reduce stress, be a protective factor against developing depression and anxiety, buffer against negative thinking, increase psychological resilience in the face of pain and illness, and even increase quality of life of people living with health conditions. People who are compassionate with themselves also tend to engage in more health-promoting behaviors, like exercise and good nutrition—one of the reasons why self-compassion predicts better physical health and fewer physical symptoms.

Amazingly, changing that negative inner voice to one of loving-kindness can affect how you *physically feel*. Pain and health experts agree: self-compassion can not only change your mood, it can change your health.

How to Do It

To do this exercise, imagine your most compassionate friend or family member. Recall the things he says and list his kind, empathic messages. Then, in moments of pain, self-criticism, or suffering, invite him into your head. Imagine his face and tone of voice, and say these compassionate things to yourself just the way he would. Alternatively, you can think of a suffering friend or family member, and consider what you'd say to him or her. Then replace your critical negative thoughts with compassionate statements full of kindness, empathy, and self-love. It may feel strange to speak kindly to yourself at first—it often does. That's because we're used to hearing our loud, beastly Pain Voices and inner critics. Change the channel and try self-compassion instead. It's important to take care of yourself in the same way (if not better than!) your friends and family would. You deserve all the tenderness you can get.

Your most compassionate friend or family member: _____

Three things that person might say to you if you were miserable or in pain:

Examples:

1. My love, I'm so sorry you're having such a hard day. You've been suffering and you don't deserve this.

2. I know you're in a lot of pain and I want you to know that I'm here for you. What can I do to help you feel better?

3. No matter what happens, I've got your back. You're never alone.

Your Examples:

1. _____
2. _____
3. _____

Think of someone you care about who's suffering. Write down his/her name:

_____

What are three things you've said, or would say, to this person to express compassion and ease his or her suffering?

1. _____
2. _____
3. _____

Now set aside five minutes and turn off your screens. Stand in front of a mirror with this page. Read aloud the compassionate messages that you've given loved ones, and that loved ones have given you. Looking at yourself in the mirror, allow these messages to sink in.

How did this feel? Note physical and emotional reactions:

_____

_____

List three triggering situations in which you hear your Pain Voice or inner critic. These are the situations in which you'll need to use your Compassionate Voice.

Examples:

1. Looking in the mirror while getting dressed.

2. During a pain flare.

3. After a conversation with my mother.

Your Examples:

1. _____
2. _____
3. _____

Prepare for future triggers by practicing Compassionate Voice. Write out what she sounds like once a day; then rehearse in the mirror. To expand your list of compassionate statements, write down the nurturing, kind things you hear yourself saying to friends and family, loving and sympathetic phrases you overhear being said to others, and even the sweet things you say to your pet. Just as with coping statements, the more you practice Compassionate Voice, the louder, stronger, and easier to access he'll get.

Your Brain Hears Everything Your Mouth Says

You may think the things you say aren't very important. But language matters, because *your brain hears everything your mouth says*. The words you say aloud are transmitted from your mouth up to your ears, then sent up to your brain for processing. So every time you say things like, "I'll never get better,"

"I can't do this," or "I'll never run again," your brain hears this and *it believes you!* For this reason, it's very important to pay attention to the words you choose.

Language Matters: Choosing Your Words

1. Give pain less airtime. Pop quiz: What does your brain's prefrontal cortex do every time you talk about pain? Answer: It turns up the pain dial, amplifying *pain*. Neuroscience tells us that focusing attention on pain actually makes us hurt more and feel *worse*, not better. Constant pain-talk requires your brain to focus on pain's distorted thoughts and words, giving Pain Voice extra airtime and more power.

To be clear, this doesn't mean you should never talk about pain or illness. Your suffering is real, and it's important to talk about it and get support. But be mindful of pain-talk—when, how much, and with whom. Take power back by giving pain *less airtime* instead of more, shifting attention and changing language.

> *After three failed back surgeries, Jeremiah experienced such terrible pain in his back and legs that he required a wheelchair. A former computer engineer, he was unable to work or effectively care for himself, so he lived with his sister and nephews. To distract and self-soothe, he wrote code on his laptop. One Saturday, Jeremiah was outside coding. He was enjoying it so much that he'd stopped noticing how badly his legs and back were aching. From the house, his sister called, "On a scale of 0 to 10, how high is your pain today?" In that moment, the smile disappeared from Jeremiah's face and his back stiffened. All of his attention went shooting back to the pain in his body. He hugged his legs with both arms and noticed that they were aching. "I think it was a 3 before," he said, "but now it's a 7."*

2. Use the word "yet." "Yet" reminds your brain that there's hope for the future. This is a great strategy to use to defend against Pain Voice, which constantly tells you that the way things are now is the way they're going to be forever. For example, instead of, "I don't take care of myself the way I keep saying I will," replace this with "I don't take care of myself the way I intend to *yet*." Instead of "I'll never play ball with my kids again," try "I can't play ball with my kids *yet*." Instead of "I haven't found the solution to this pain problem and I never will," practice saying "I haven't found the solution to this pain problem *yet*." This reminds your brain that the way things are now is *not* necessarily the way they'll always be, and asserts the possibility of change.

3. End negative expectations. It's easy to get trapped into talking about a life with pain as though negative outcomes were inevitable. Allow your brain to believe that life will improve, even if you have to fake it at first. Don't just imagine it—*expect* it. To do this, replace the word "if" with the word "when." For example, instead of "*If* I ever dance again…" try saying "*When* I feel well enough to dance" or "*When* this pain episode is over." Take out mights and maybes. Instead of "I might try walking today," say "I *will* walk for ten minutes today and see how I feel." You're more likely to actually and successfully do the things you tell yourself you can do, even if they're hard, if you set a *positive expectation*. Positive expectations may not always feel realistic, but you aren't doing yourself any favors by believing Pain Voice's negative predictions. Imagining positive outcomes can change your behaviors in ways that make them more likely to actually occur! Give yourself hope—it's one of the most important gifts there is.

Complete the following sentences:

Two things I'll do when my pain is more manageable:

1. _____

2. _____

By this time next year, I picture myself being able to:

_____

_____

_____

4. Leave past pain where it belongs: in the past. Those of us with chronic pain often ruminate about past pain episodes and predict that the next episode will be equally bad or worse. While this is normal, it can trigger feelings of dejection, anger, and hopelessness. Focusing on past medical traumas keeps your brain stuck. It can also transport you back in time, affecting both mind and body. Just as envisioning that beach in Mexico can inspire relaxation and calm, constantly replaying past pain episodes can invite fear, stress, and more pain. Imagery is a powerful tool we want to use to help, not hurt. For this reason, it's important to leave past pain episodes where they belong: in the past. To achieve this difficult task, (1) notice your language, reducing time spent ruminating about past medical issues and pain, and (2) consider working with a therapist who specializes in trauma or pain so that you can heal from the inside out.

Take Power Back from Pain

Words that commonly describe chronic pain or illness reflect powerlessness and low self-reliance. Circle any words that sound familiar:

Sick	Weak	Disabled	Powerless
Ill	Damaged	Broken	

When you say these words, do they make you feel good—like you can do anything—or bad, like you'd rather crawl under a blanket and hide? Words focusing on pain and powerlessness keep you submissive and miserable. Instead, flip that language upside down. Start using words that make you feel strong and empowered instead, like these:

Resilient	Strong	Confident	Powerful
Healthy	Competent	Capable	

If these descriptors don't feel true to you, that's okay—even expected. Pain takes away power: that's its job. This can make it hard to tap into your strengths. But healing is a process, and feeling powerless isn't permanent. *Take your power back* using powerful language, even if you have to fake it 'til you make it. Pain doesn't rule you, even if it sometimes seems to. Your strengths, abilities, and accomplishments define you more than any health condition ever could. Give them a moment to shine. Look at the following sentence examples, then complete your own:

I am *Resilient* because:

(I never stop trying and always get back up when I get knocked down.)

_____

I feel *Healthy* when I:

(go swimming at the local pool.)

_____

A time I felt *Strong* was:

(when I talked to my boss about my needs at work.)

_____

I am *Confident* about (physical attributes, skills, accomplishments...):

(my beautiful blue eyes, my ability to problem-solve in tough situations, the award I won last year.)

_____

_____

I am *Capable* because I can do the following things on my own:

(repair my car, take care of my finances, show up for my kids.)

_____

_____

What fills you with a sense of *Power?*

(when I set boundaries, boxing, building something)

1. _____

2. _____

3. _____

Gratitudes and Good Things

The "Gratitudes and Good Things" activity regulates pain by inspiring feelings of happiness and gratitude. Noticing the good things in your life, no matter how small, helps you focus on things for which you're grateful, lifting your mood and shifting your attention away from pain to things that inspire joy. This trains your brain to notice people and experiences that generate feelings of happiness, love, and safety. It also tunes you in to things that make life worth living!

Research shows that gratitude practices and positive thoughts can improve overall mood; increase your sense of meaning and purpose; reduce frustration, anger, and irritability; reduce loneliness; promote immune functioning; reduce symptoms of illness; increase ability to cope with pain; and improve overall physical health. A regular gratitude practice like this one can even change your brain pathways, rewiring your brain.

Positive thoughts and gratitudes also increase the brain's production of *serotonin* and *dopamine*, chemical messengers that regulate mood, appetite, sleep…and pain. For these reasons, the Gratitudes and Good Things activity can be a powerful addition to any pain-management plan.

How to Do It

Find a quiet place to sit where you won't be disturbed for ten to twenty minutes. Turn off all screens. Make a list of Ten Good Things for which you're grateful or that make you feel happy. These can be memories, kind things people have done for you, kind things you've done for others, a list of favorites (foods, movies, books, animals, vacations), activities you're looking forward to, people you admire, and any other good things that have happened in your life. They don't have to be big things—they can be as ordinary as your cat purring or a gooey slice of pizza. It can be something that happened this week or many years ago.

Here are my Ten Good Things:

1. Hiking in nature

2. Tortoiseshell butterflies

3. Freshly baked New York bagels

4. Childhood friendships that endure into adulthood

5. Memories of dancing with Grandpa Norman

6. Holding the door open for strangers

7. Learning about the brain

8. Bioluminescent jellyfish that make their own light

9. Bookstores with a secret door disguised as a bookshelf

10. Autumn in Vermont

Yadira's Example

Yadira was miserable. After six years of treatment, her chronic illness still caused her pain and her medications weren't working. She was irritable and moody, thinking things like, "There's nothing good in my life." She stressed about work, mortgage payments, taking care of her aging parents, and keeping her family fed. Lately it seemed that she argued with everyone; last week she argued bitterly with her father, and this week her boyfriend threatened to leave after a terrible fight. These situational and emotional triggers made her body feel worse. On a scale of 1 to 10, her pain was an 11.

When Yadira learned the Ten Good Things activity, she started paying attention to the small things in her life that made her less miserable, even if only briefly—like pancakes for dinner and warm laundry from the dryer. For the next week, she listed ten things every day that made her feel grateful and good. When she did this, Yadira noticed that, while it didn't solve her problems or cure her illness, her mood lifted and attention shifted, and she had space to focus on some of the good things in her life.

After two weeks, Yadira framed her favorite "Top Twenty" Things, decorated the frame, and hung it next to her bed. She loved looking at it, and noticed that, on the days she wrote Good Things, her pain was easier to bear.

Allow yourself to write Ten Good Things every day, whether they're gratitudes, enjoyable memories, or daily observations. Carry a notebook or leave one next to your bed. Establish a regular time to practice writing, like first thing in the morning or just before bed, so that you get into a routine. Notice how this practice makes you feel. To generate Good Things, start by finishing the following sentences:

I feel grateful for…

_____

_____

Something kind I did for someone was…

_____

Something kind someone did for me was…

_____

The best vacation I ever took was…

_____

One of my favorite memories is…

_____

_____

_____

Three of my favorite things are:

1. _____

2. _____

3. _____

Three things that made me happy as a child were:

1. _____

2. _____

3. _____

Something that made me happy recently was…

_____

_____

YOUR TEN GOOD THINGS

Now make today's list. These can be sourced from the answers you generated above, or ideas they inspired.

1. _____

2. _____

3. _____

4. _____

5. _____

6. _____

7. _____

8. _____

9. _____

10. _____

How did this practice make you feel, physically and emotionally?

_____

_____

_____

Commit to writing Ten Good Things each day. When and where will you practice? (*Example: On the couch every night at 10 p.m.*)

_____

A blank copy of this exercise can be found at http://www.newharbinger.com/46448.

Imagine a Miracle

Another cognitive strategy for coping with pain is to *imagine a miracle*. Use your powerful brain to imagine a future free of struggle with pain and illness, in which you're living a happy, healthy life. This exercise helps overcome hopelessness by looking beyond the symptoms and obstacles keeping you stuck, and by inspiring you to think about goals and how you'll achieve them. Imagining a miracle can be a transformative road map to health and healing.

How to Do It

Sit somewhere calm and quiet where you won't be disturbed. Turn off your screens and put them away. Picture yourself five years from now. Imagine that a miracle has occurred and you are healed. You've overcome pain and illness. You're happy, active, successful, and fulfilled. You're wherever you dream of being, doing whatever you dream of doing, with whomever you dream of doing it with. You're healthy and strong, and have achieved your dreams. After envisioning this miracle, read Henry's answers to the following questions. Then answer the questions on your own in the space provided.

You wake up without any pain or illness. What's the first thing you do?

When I realize I have no pain, I leap out of bed and throw away my leg brace. I run up and down the stairs simply because I can, then call my family, friends, and everyone I know to tell them the news. I put on my sneakers, drive to the ocean with my dog, and take him for a long run on the beach.

How does it feel to be without pain or illness?

It feels amazing. I feel lighter. I use my legs as much as I want. I smile a lot. I talk to everyone.

How do you spend your time (work and play)?

I live in Mexico and teach children. I have a huge community of family and friends and speak fluent Spanish. I've learned to make chilaquiles and banana bread. On weekends I travel around the country, exploring historical sites and meeting people. I run on the beach and kayak every chance I get.

Five years ago, you were struggling with pain and illness. What steps did you take to get from there to here?

Five years ago, I developed complex regional pain syndrome (CRPS) and couldn't walk. I'd planned to spend a year teaching in Mexico, but the program wouldn't admit me because of my health. I set a goal to get strong enough to walk with just one crutch by March. I went to physical therapy, did pacing and desensitization exercises, and learned CBT strategies to manage pain. When my mood started improving, I had more motivation and energy. By March I was strong enough to walk with one crutch; then without any by June. Since the Mexico program demanded I be able to run, I used pacing to start jogging. It took some time, but eventually I was able to run again. I went to Mexico to teach and it changed my life. This is my calling. Now I am fit, active, doing what I love, and I feel amazing.

_____

_____

_____

_____

_____

_____

What qualities do you have that enabled you to take these steps?

Tenacity, resilience, patience, and persistence.

_____

_____

What helped the most?

Three things: (1) Finding healthcare providers I liked and trusted. (2) Identifying a motivating, aspirational goal: teach in Mexico for a year. (3) Picking an end goal and a starting point. End goal = walk without crutches by summer. Starting point = go to physical therapy daily and

CBT weekly, and set small, achievable objectives. Every successful baby step gave me momentum to continue toward the next small goal.

What obstacles did you face as you healed, and how did you overcome them?

Fear of pain was the biggest obstacle. CRPS treatment required me to use my painful leg—but I was scared to walk, so I avoided it. The longer I avoided movement, the worse my pain got and the less progress I made. When I identified the meaningful goal of teaching in Mexico, my motivation increased. I used the skills I learned in CBT and physical therapy to take one small step at a time, and accepted support from my providers, family, and friends. It gave me the strength I needed to persist in the face of pain. I was determined to prove I could do it, and I did.

How does it feel to imagine a miracle? How can you use this technique to move your life one step forward?

What three small actions can you take NOW to move you closer to your goal?

1. _____

2. _____

3. _____

Conclusion

There's a real, biological connection between the thoughts in your head and the sensations in your body. Pain Voice generates anxious, catastrophic, negative thoughts that amplify pain and keep you feeling low. Pain Voice is powerful, but not more powerful than you. Because cognitive factors influence pain processing, transforming thoughts can transform pain. Wise Voice, coping thoughts, self-compassion, going gray, shifting attention, changing language, noticing gratitudes and good things, and imagining miracles can help you take your power back. In the next chapter, you'll learn how lifestyle factors like sleep, nutrition, exercise, and social support can also turn down your pain dial!

CHAPTER 7

Lifestyle Tips for Pain Management

Why do doctors always ask about lifestyle decisions like sleep, nutrition, and exercise? Our daily choices and way of life significantly affect how we feel. In this chapter we'll look at the ways our behavioral patterns impact health and pain.

Brains Love Balance

Your body craves *homeostasis*, or balance. When your body is off-balance, you're more prone to sickness and pain. Your body is strongest and happiest when you drink enough water, keep blood sugar steady, sleep consistently every night, get sunlight, use your muscles, and aren't too sedentary. Not too little of anything, and not too much.

Your brain helps you maintain homeostasis by sending signals that something isn't right. For example, hunger pangs and headaches are signals that you're low on fuel and need to eat. Drowsiness and irritability are signals that you need more sleep. When a room gets too hot, your body instructs you to shed that sweater! Your body has many ways of telling you that something's off-balance—including physical symptoms like pain.

Being off-balance is a trigger for pain.

To prevent and cope with pain flares, make a *homeostasis plan:*

- Eat three healthy *meals* each day.

- Maintain good *sleep hygiene.*

- Drink *water* throughout the day.

- *Move* and exercise daily to keep bones, brain, and muscles strong.

- Go outside, enjoy *nature,* and get *sunlight.*

- Spend time alone and time with *community.*

In this chapter, we'll cover important lifestyle decisions. Lets start with sleep, since you do it every night.

Sleep Better to Feel Better

Sleep plays an important role in pain and illness. Sleep is a time of rest and repair, but when you're sick and in pain, your sleep cycle is easily thrown off-balance and homeostasis is disrupted. Poor sleep at night leads to sleeping late and taking naps. Daytime sleep makes it even harder to sleep at night. Lying in bed awake for hours with insomnia triggers frustration, anxiety, and worry about your inability to sleep, making it even *harder* to sleep—and turns up the pain dial. This leads to yet another night of poor rest, then sleep catchup the next day...and around and around the cycle goes.

Chronic pain can trigger various sleep issues: trouble falling asleep, irregular sleep patterns, nighttime awakenings, and poor sleep quality. Lack of sleep and insomnia are then associated with increased pain and symptoms. Moreover, poor sleep can affect all aspects of your life, from cognitive functioning to physical performance to completion of tasks. For these reasons, developing healthy sleep habits is an important part of your recovery.

Human beings are *diurnal,* which means our brains are programmed to be alert and awake when the sun is shining, and to shut down and sleep at night. This is distinct from *nocturnal* animals, like owls and bats, whose brains are programmed to sleep during the day and wake at night.

Your sleep cycle is regulated by a brain structure called the *suprachiasmatic nucleus* (SCN). The SCN is your built-in alarm clock. It influences your body's twenty-four-hour rhythms—when you get hungry, when you feel alert and active, and when you crash and need sleep. The SCN is programmed by sunlight, which means that you can "set" your SCN like you set your alarm clock at night. This is in part due to a brain chemical called *melatonin,* which regulates your sleep–wake cycle. This cycle allows your body to repair and refresh, and keeps you in sync with the sun and the outside world.

If you're experiencing sleep difficulties, help is available. The American College of Physicians recommends trying CBT-I (Cognitive Behavioral Therapy for Insomnia) *before* using sleep medications like trazodone, Ambien, benzodiazepines, melatonin, or other sleep aids, because these chemicals can disrupt your natural rhythms. Some medications also have addictive properties, leading to a reliance on them to fall asleep. Physicians therefore recommend behavioral interventions as the first-line treatment for chronic insomnia and sleep issues. CBT-I incorporates sleep hygiene techniques like the ones in this book with other cognitive and behavioral strategies. Unlike pills, these interventions can address common underlying causes of insomnia—like pain or anxiety—rather than just the symptoms. CBT-I and sleep hygiene programs are scientifically-supported treatments for insomnia and other sleep issues, and have the added benefit of having zero side effects and no risk of addiction. In short: you have nothing to lose!

To find a provider, visit the Society of Behavioral Sleep Medicine at www.behavioralsleep.org (enter your location under "provider search") or try the International Directory of CBT-I Providers (www.cbti.directory). You can also search online for a "CBT-I provider near me."

Sleep Tracking

Track your sleep habits for a week and record them here. Download blank forms at http://www .newharbinger.com/46448. Make sure to include the use of sleep medications and other substances. This assessment will help determine what interventions will be most useful.

Sleep Tracker

	Example	Mon.	Tues.	Wed.	Thurs.	Fri.	Sat.	Sun.
Bedtime	11 p.m.							
Wake time	7 a.m.							
Number and length of naps	1 nap, 45 minutes							
Insomnia?	Yes							
Night awakenings?	Yes, 2							
Total time spent in bed	8.5 hours							
Total hours of sleep	4.5 hours							
Sleep medications?	Yes, trazodone 150 mg							
Substances (drugs/alcohol)?	Yes, 2 glasses of wine							

Sleep Hygiene

Use *sleep hygiene* to recover from pain-related sleep deprivation and establish healthier sleep practices. These tips and behavior changes can reduce insomnia, minimize night awakenings, and target other sleep issues. For quick improvement, try all of them consistently starting tonight; or implement them two at a time, folding in a few new tips each week. The more you make sleep hygiene a regular nightly habit, the quicker your brain will adjust and the better your sleep is likely to get. Keeping old habits will only lead to continued poor sleep.

- **Get into bed only when sleepy.** "Tired" and "sleepy" are not the same. You may feel fatigued and tired after a long day, but still not be sleepy enough to fall asleep. Getting in bed before you're sleepy leads to lying there, frustrated and awake.

- **Create a comfortable sleep environment.** Make your room dark, cool, and quiet. Use a white-noise machine or fan to keep your bedroom peaceful. Put up curtains so street lights don't keep you up at bedtime and sunlight doesn't wake you before wake time. Temperature is also important: have you ever noticed how hard it is to fall asleep on hot summer nights? Our body temperature naturally drops at night, and we sleep better in cool environments.

- **Use your bed only for sleep.** Find another comfortable place to watch TV, read, or text. Train your brain to associate bed *exclusively* with sleep. Why? Your brain quickly learns relationships between things. If you lie in bed awake, your brain will associate "bed" with "wakefulness." However, if you use your bed only for sleep, your brain will learn that "bed" = "unconscious and drooling"!

- **Don't check the time.** Watching the clock only increases stress and anxiety: *It's 3 a.m., I won't be able to function tomorrow!* The more anxious you get, the *less* likely you are to fall asleep—so cover your clocks and keep your phone in another room or out of sight.

- **Get out of bed after twenty minutes.** If you can't fall asleep, don't lie in bed worrying. Get out of bed after approximately twenty minutes (no need to check the clock!) and do something calming: read a book on the couch, or listen to relaxing music in a comfy chair. Then get back into bed when you're sleepy. Why? The longer you lie in bed stressed about not sleeping, the more activated your body gets. The more activated and anxious you are, the less likely you are to sleep! Lying awake in bed for long periods also teaches your brain to associate bed with anxious wakefulness rather than relaxed sleepiness.

- **Have calming, soothing activities ready.** When you can't sleep, don't search for something to do. Keep a book, magazine, or headphones in a comfortable and accessible place, like next to your couch. Make sure to choose activities that are relaxing—like drawing or reading—rather than activating, like watching the news. Get an old-school, inexpensive MP3 player or streaming device that doesn't have a clock so that you can listen to music without stressing about the time.

- **Set a sleep time and wake time.** Brains love routine. Waking up and falling asleep at the same time every day sets your SCN (biological clock). The earlier you wake up, the earlier you'll be able to fall asleep. Consistent sleep and wake times are crucial, *especially* if you're not waking up for work in the morning—otherwise, your biological clock will fall out of sync. Because your body craves balance, your brain is happiest when it has a routine—so turn it "off" and "on" at the same time every day.

- **Get exposure to sunlight.** First thing in the morning, open your curtains and get sunlight or step outside. Your SCN, which triggers the release of "sleep" chemicals in the dark, breaks down these chemicals to signal "wake" in the light. This sets your biological clock and reminds your brain that light = wake, and dark = sleep.

- **Limit or eliminate naps.** As tempting as naps are, especially when you're exhausted and in pain, teach your brain that "sleep" happens at night, and "awake" happens during the day. Napping partially satisfies sleep needs, which reduces your need to sleep at night—making it more likely that you'll experience difficulty falling and staying asleep. If you must nap, limit naps to fifteen or twenty minutes and stick to earlier in the day rather than later. For better sleep, restrict sleep to nighttime only.

- **Establish a relaxing pre-bedtime routine.** Before bed, take a hot bath, read, or do relaxation exercises or meditations. Avoid work, screens, news reports, arguments, stimulating activities, or anything stressful. Make a list of relaxing, pre-bedtime activities you can try. Once you get into a nightly rhythm, these activities will start cueing your brain that it's time to start shutting down.

- **Don't take your problems to bed.** Do you ever lie in bed chewing over problems and worrying about things you need to do? Do you think about world news, or try to solve all of your problems? Bedtime is a terrible time to worry and problem-solve. Pick a "worry time" earlier in the day and write down concerns, plans, and to-dos. Then, at night, remind yourself that you'll log more "worry time" tomorrow to give your concerns a place to go.

- **Exercise.** Exercise regulates brain chemistry and helps your body feel tired. It also eats up stress hormones like adrenaline produced during the day that keep you activated.

Exercise earlier in the day and avoid exercising in the evening so that your body stays relaxed and cool for bedtime.

- **Reduce fluids before bedtime.** Nobody likes getting in and out of bed seven times a night to use the bathroom. The urge to go can interrupt healthy sleep cycles.

- **Avoid caffeine and alcohol.** These substances interfere with natural sleep–wake signals: caffeine artificially speeds you up, and alcohol artificially slows you down. Both can disrupt your biological rhythms. If you're already having trouble sleeping, these substances will only get in the way of tuning in to your natural sleep signals. Using substances to artificially speed up and slow down are surefire ways to keep your sleep cycle dysregulated.

- **Avoid sugar and big meals before bed.** Sugar and food are fuel that prepare your body for action. Teach your brain that nighttime is for slowing down, not revving up.

- **Avoid sleeping in more than two hours on weekends.** It's delightful to catch up on sleep, but what happens when your body gets used to staying up 'til 1 a.m. and sleeping late on Saturday and Sunday? By Sunday night, you can't fall asleep until late, so Monday morning feels even more miserable. This pattern leads to sleep deprivation, exhaustion, and increased pain. Limit extra weekend sleep to a couple hours max.

- **Avoid sleeping with pets if you have sleep difficulties.** They're cute, comforting, and fuzzy, it's true—but they also snore, kick, lick your face, and climb in and out of bed—which disturbs your sleep. No wonder you're so tired in the morning!

- **Limit screens before bed.** As hard as it is, try to limit screen time to a few hours per day. Turn off screens a few hours before bed and do something else (read, draw, talk) instead. Remove screens from your bedroom at night: they're too tempting. Leave them in a basket in the kitchen or living room, and retrieve them at breakfast. If you use your phone as an alarm, consider getting a boring, basic alarm clock for your bedroom instead. Why? Blue light from screens suppresses melatonin, the brain chemical that regulates sleep. Low melatonin = less likely to fall asleep. Screens also stimulate your brain, providing sensory overload during a time when you should be helping your brain shut down. Lastly, screens activate your sympathetic nervous system—and stress hormones like adrenaline are terrible for sleep. Brainstorm calming activities that don't involve screens, like the ones in this book.

- **After a tough night, avoid sleeping in.** After a night of poor sleep, morning exhaustion naturally leads to the urge to sleep late. However, sleeping in reduces "sleep pressure," or the drive to sleep that builds up over the course of the day. Higher sleep pressure = more likely to sleep. The longer you sleep in, the *less* likely you are to get sleepy at a reasonable time the following night. Research shows that waking early—especially after a bad night—helps the sleep cycle return to normal. Have you ever noticed that people who wake at 4 a.m. for work or have newborns rarely seem to have insomnia? As hard as it is, resist the urge to sleep in.

- **Don't rearrange your life around sleep.** As difficult and counterintuitive as this may be, *continue with life as usual.* Sleep difficulties often stem from, and inevitably trigger, anxiety. Anxiety obnoxiously demands that you reorganize your life around it, but doing so only gives anxiety more power. Moreover, every time you do something differently, you're reminded of sleep issues—which increases anxiety. For this reason, don't rearrange your schedule or do things differently because of sleep issues. Sleep anxiety doesn't get to be in charge of your life—you do. Follow all of these sleep hygiene tips, and you'll no longer need to rearrange your life around sleep.

Your Sleep Hygiene Plan

Want results fast? Use all of these tips tonight, every single one. If you want to go slowly and need a place to start, pick two or three tips to try this week and add two more next week. Changing habits is hard and doesn't happen overnight. It's like building a muscle—it takes practice and time. Try a few and see how it goes!

Which three sleep hygiene strategies will you try this week? If you're ready to try all, write "All."

1. _____

2. _____

3. _____

Daily bedtime goal this week: _____ p.m.

Daily wake time goal: _____ a.m.

How will you stick to these sleep times? (*set two alarms, ask my spouse to hold me accountable*)

_____

Three relaxing, nonscreen activities for your pre-bedtime routine (*take a hot bath, read a magazine, listen to a body scan*):

1. _____
2. _____
3. _____

Where you'll go if you can't fall asleep and need to get out of bed (*living room couch, bedroom chair*):

_____

Relaxing activities you'll have ready in case you can't sleep (*headphones and music, nature magazine*):

_____

_____

Ideas for not looking at clocks (*turn bedside clock around, leave phone in kitchen*):

_____

Where you'll store screens before bed (*kitchen drawer, basket by the door*):

_____

One way you've been rearranging your life around sleep (*don't go out after 8 p.m., ask spouse to manage the kids at bedtime*):

_____

_____

How will you plan to resume normal behavior? (*I'll make plans to stay out with friends later than 8 p.m. on Saturday.*)

_____

Exercise and the Brain

"Why are people always telling me to exercise?"

It can be annoying to hear doctor after doctor tell you to exercise—especially when you're in pain. As frustrating as it is, here's why they insist: Studies show that exercise increases energy and reduces fatigue among people with chronic pain and illness; stimulates muscle, tissue, and bone repair; improves joint function; reduces risk of developing chronic illnesses; improves sleep; and can reduce pain. There's more: exercise helps your blood circulate (which provides your body with oxygen to support tissue repair), facilitates healing, and boosts immune functioning. It can also bolster self-esteem, decrease and prevent stress and anxiety, lift mood to reduce depression, and turn down the pain dial.

On the flip side, lack of movement leads to reduced immune functioning; stiffness, muscle tension, and muscle atrophy; feeling weak and lethargic; decreased motivation; and increased and prolonged pain. Because of this, being sedentary—not exercising—is one of the biggest risk factors for developing lifelong chronic pain and illness. (All this research makes me want to go for a walk!)

In addition to healing your body, movement and exercise change…wait for it…your brain. (Surprise!) *Exercise rewires your pain system*, lowering the pain alarm and stimulating the production of brain chemicals that are part of the pain-relief response, including:

- *Serotonin*—regulates mood and other functions. When serotonin goes up, mood generally goes up and pain volume goes down. Most commonly prescribed antidepressants and anti-anxiety medications target serotonin.

- *Dopamine*—transmits feelings of pleasure and reward to turn down your pain dial.

- *Endorphins*—your body's natural painkillers. Endorphins muffle pain. Many pain medications actually imitate the effects of endorphins! (Isn't it impressive that your body created them first?)

In addition to regulating neurotransmitters, exercise also eats up stress hormones like adrenaline and cortisol that are released during fight-or-flight, thereby promoting relaxation and healing. It may seem counterintuitive, but when you're chronically ill or in pain, it's *especially* important to exercise. This doesn't mean you should immediately resume the exercise routines you had before your pain started. Rather, if you've been inactive for weeks or months, try to resume activity slowly. Try physical therapy and occupational therapy for tips, guidance, and support. Use your pacing plan from chapter 3! Take a daily walk, attend a swim class, or try yoga, which combines stretching, strength training, and mindful body awareness. Think about ways you most enjoy moving your body even if you have some pain.

Top Ten Physical Activities for Chronic Pain

It can be hard to move when you hurt. Identifying a form of physical activity that feels manageable is therefore very important. Review the list of options below and choose at least one you're willing to try. Then develop a pacing plan to help you get started. Many of these can be done in the comfort of your own home. Even trying is a victory!

1. **Walk outdoors:** Low impact, easily accessible, strengthens body, lubricates joints, exposure to sunlight and nature.

2. **Stretch:** Improves range of motion and flexibility, stimulates blood flow and full-body relaxation.

3. **Swim:** Very low impact, whole-body fitness, joint-friendly, strengthens muscles while increasing endurance.

4. **Yoga:** A form of mindful movement that integrates stretching, breathing, meditation, body awareness, and strengthening.

5. **Tai Chi:** Low impact, stimulates blood flow, can reduce stress and worry, integrates mind and body.

6. **Strength training:** Targets specific muscle groups using light weights and isometrics to increase strength and fitness.

7. **Dance:** Facilitates self-expression (teakettling!); stimulates circulation while exercising core, legs, and arms; decreases fear of movement; increases motivation to move.

8. **Stationary bike:** Low impact, strengthens leg and heart muscles.

9. **Walk on a treadmill or in a pool:** Low impact, improves blood flow, strengthens muscles and cardiovascular system, offers control of pace and incline.

10. **Sex:** Yes, really. Sex not only requires cardio work and endurance, it also triggers the release of endorphins—your brain's natural painkillers. Get out of breath, desensitize your brain, and use your body!

Building an Exercise Hierarchy

As with pacing for activities, it's important to resume exercise slowly and gradually so that your brain and body have a chance to adjust. The boom-and-bust cycle of over- and underdoing it simply doesn't work. Create a plan to resume exercise by first identifying your ultimate goal (for example, resume rock climbing), then building a hierarchy of action steps required to get there, from smallest to largest. Ask yourself: What muscles do I need to strengthen before I can do this activity? How much endurance is required and how do I build that up? Include steps that will help you get back into the habit of exercising. Then put all the action steps in your Exercise Hierarchy, as Matt did here. Each goal should build on the previous one, so that when you reach the end of your hierarchy, you're able to do all the activities required to meet your goal. Your hierarchy can have as few or as many steps as you like, as long as it's realistic for *you*. You can download a blank copy at http://www .newharbinger.com/46448.

Matt's Exercise Hierarchy

Ultimate exercise goal: Resume rock climbing	
Step 1: Get back into the habit of going to the climbing gym.	Action: Go to gym and just watch for 1 week. Sit with friends and tell them my intent to return.
Step 2: Strengthen upper body.	Action: 15 pull-ups a day for 1 week + back exercises.
Step 3: Increase endurance and lung capacity.	Action: Walk 15 minutes daily for 2 weeks + continue strengthening exercises.
Step 4: Get reacquainted with the climbing wall.	Action: Climb an easy route for 10 minutes 3 days this week (Mon, Wed, Sat).
Step 5: Solve simple boulder problem.	Action: Ask climbing partner to meet me at the gym on Sunday for support. Solve one 30-minute boulder problem.

Your Exercise Hierarchy

Ultimate exercise goal:	
Step 1:	Action:
Step 2:	Action:
Step 3:	Action:
Step 4:	Action:
Step 5:	Action:

Your Exercise Plan

1. State your ultimate exercise goal. (*Example: Swim for 30 minutes daily.*)

    _____

    _____

2. What exercise or movement goals would you like to commit to this week? (*Example: Register for water aerobics class, ride stationary bike for 10 minutes*)

    _____

    _____

3. When and where will you implement this plan? (*Example: Wednesday morning, today after lunch*)

    _____

    _____

4. Select an "accountability partner." Who will help you keep this commitment and achieve your goal?

    _____

    _____

5. How can you make movement a regular habit? (*Example: Sign up for weekly class to gain momentum, go to the gym with Sara every Friday*)

    _____

    _____

6. When will you start your Exercise Hierarchy?

    _____

    _____

Sunlight and Nature Are Medicines

Pain and illness work together to keep you stuck indoors without exercise, hobbies, social activity, or sunlight. It's time to fight back! Exposure to sunlight is critical for health: sunshine regulates sleep and wake cycles, increases serotonin to improve mood, and stimulates the production of vitamin D—a vitamin critical for physical strength and healthy functioning. According to scientific studies, sunlight and vitamin D may also provide protection against illnesses such as rheumatoid arthritis, asthma, and infectious diseases.

Research also suggests that nature—the sight of green trees, the smell of pinecones and fresh-cut grass, the sounds of crickets and rainfall—can positively impact mood, stress, memory, attention, concentration, health, and ability to cope with pain. If you've ever noticed that candle companies, sports drinks, and beauty products rely on nature for marketing, our positive association with nature is the reason why. Research indicates that most of us are sunlight- and nature-deprived and crave reconnection. So whenever you schedule activities or exercise, plan social events, or practice coping strategies, consider going outside. *Sunlight and nature are medicines!*

What are three ways you can add more nature to your life?

1. _____

2. _____

3. _____

One activity you can do outside today:

_____

Nutrition and Health: Eat Better to Feel Better

Food is your body's fuel source, like gas in a car. But food doesn't just give you energy: good nutrition is crucial for good health. Food contains nutrients like vitamins and minerals that help your body run smoothly, like a machine. For example, calcium, a mineral found in dairy products, helps strengthen and repair bones, facilitates immune functioning, helps blood clot, and allows brain cells to communicate. Without calcium, your brain and body simply wouldn't function.

Sometimes pain leads to eating less, skipping meals, or developing unhealthy eating habits. This can cause exhaustion, fatigue, headaches, body aches, and more pain. It can also lead to *vitamin or mineral deficiencies*, meaning that your body is getting fewer nutrients than it needs. When you are deficient, your body is less able to battle pain and health issues. Deficiencies also prevent your immune system from functioning properly, increasing susceptibility to illness and making it harder for your body to fight off infections. *Being vitamin and mineral deficient can not only make you sick, but also prevent you from getting well.*

Food, or lack of it, can also affect mood. Have you ever been "hangry," or so hungry that you became irritable and angry? This is your body telling you that you're out of balance and need food! However, not all foods are created equal: some foods are healthier, while others are less healthy. Processed foods high in sugar and preservatives, like fast food, soda, and sugar cereals, have been shown to exacerbate inflammation, trigger headaches, and contribute to heart disease and obesity. There's some evidence that food additives and chemicals like aspartame (NutraSweet) and sucralose (Splenda), commonly found in diet foods and diet drinks, are associated with pain and increased risk of cancer. Similarly, MSG, a flavor enhancer commonly found in canned foods and Chinese restaurants, may be associated with migraines and headaches.

This doesn't mean you should stop eating all your favorite foods! No way. It simply means you need to find a good balance. Not too much food and not too little; not too many rich, fatty, sweet foods, and not too much deprivation. What you put into your body determines what you get out of your body.

Nutrition for Pain

When you're sick or in pain, it's important to eat a variety of fresh, whole foods, including fruits, vegetables, whole grains, dairy products, lean proteins, and healthy fats. Consider avoiding or dialing back on caffeine (a stimulant that amplifies your body's stress response), alcohol (a depressant that disrupts sleep and can negatively affect liver, brain, and other organs), heavy meals late at night, diet foods and drinks full of chemicals, and processed foods with ingredients you can't pronounce.

Here are some healthy foods that can promote healing. Optimize your body's ability to fight pain, and circle a few you're willing to try!

- Fruit: red grapes, blueberries, strawberries, apples, oranges, pears, cherries, bananas

- Vegetables: leafy greens, carrots, avocados, beets, broccoli, Brussels sprouts, cabbage, cauliflower, kale

- Nuts: walnuts, almonds, pecans, peanuts

- Seeds: pumpkin, sunflower, and so on

- Whole grains: brown rice, lentils, oatmeal, quinoa, couscous, whole wheat bread, whole grain pasta, popcorn

- Black beans

- Eggs

- Dairy: milk, yogurt, cheese

- Fish: salmon, cod, tuna, trout, mackerel, herring, sardines

- Chicken soup (ask Grandma for her recipe!)

- Antioxidant tea (such as green tea)

- Ginger

- Olive oil

Your Nutrition Plan

Three healthy foods you'll add to your diet this week:

1. _____

2. _____

3. _____

Two unhealthy foods you'll eat less of:

1. _____

2. _____

Your plan to ensure three healthy meals a day (*for example: set a "meal alarm," share your nutrition plan with your family, shop for groceries on the list*):

_____

_____

Three ideas for integrating healthy foods into meals (*for example: add fruit to breakfast, use olive oil instead of butter, switch to whole grain bread for lunch, add a vegetable side dish at dinner, snack on nuts instead of cookies*):

_____

_____

Hydration Is Medicine

Drinking enough water, or *hydrating*, is an often overlooked and important part of any good pain-management plan. Water flushes toxins from your system, lubricates joints, reduces joint pain, and prevents and stops muscle cramps. Water is required for the production of hormones and neurotransmitters, facilitates temperature regulation via sweating and respiration, flushes body waste, helps deliver oxygen to all your body parts, and allows your cells to grow and survive. Staying hydrated can also boost energy levels, bolster your immune system, prevent headaches and body pain, and help with alertness and focus. It's typically recommended that you drink eight or more glasses of water each day, but most of us don't drink enough.

How does your body feel when you're dehydrated?

_____

What are two ways you can make sure to drink more water this week? (*for example: carry a water bottle to work, drink an extra glass at every meal, leave a pitcher by the TV*)

1. _____

2. _____

Social Medicine

What do social factors have to do with your back pain or your cancer diagnosis? Science tells us that social factors play a critical role in pain—so much so that they are one-third of this biopsychosocial issue.

Consider this: What's the worst punishment you can give a human being? It isn't Thanksgiving traffic or even prison (but good guess). If you misbehave in prison, you're put in solitary confinement—isolated in a room by yourself, cut off from all contact and communication. What does it say about humans that the worst punishment you can give us is to isolate us from others?

Humans are biologically programmed to be social, and healthy functioning depends on it. To survive the wilderness when we were hunters and gatherers, we needed to collaborate, cooperate, and care for one another in order to secure food, water, and shelter. Having more people around provided safety from predators and protected the tribe. In fact, social behavior is so critical for survival that your brain evolved a system to reward you for it: when you're social, your brain releases *oxytocin, serotonin,* and *dopamine*: neurotransmitters that transmit feelings of happiness, connectedness, reward, and pleasure. Your brain also releases *endorphins*—your body's homemade painkillers.

Chances are high you've already experienced some of the social components of pain without even realizing it. It's that time you were sick with the flu as a child, and your mom rubbed your back and told you everything was going to be okay—and you felt a little better. It's when sharing terrible news with loved ones seems to cut the burden in half. It's the way hope swells and your spirits rise when a friend says, "You're not alone." It's discovering a group of people with the same diagnosis, who are enduring similar difficulties, and sharing stories. It's when friends bring you food or someone holds your hand. It's the comfort of having a caring, compassionate treatment team in your corner.

People coping with chronic pain are often cut off from friends and peers, and feel left out or left behind. When we're socially isolated, serotonin and dopamine levels plummet, and we may become anxious, lonely, and depressed—negative mood states that increase pain volume. In fact, the pain of isolation and social rejection is processed by the same parts of the brain as physical pain. *Being lonely hurts.*

Social isolation also triggers release of the stress hormone *cortisol*, weakening your immune system and triggering inflammation. Moreover, research shows that loneliness and isolation can increase likelihood of illness and death in the elderly. It's therefore important for your *physical* health to take care of your *social* health!

The social domain of pain also includes cultural, socioeconomic, and environmental factors. Low income, lack of access to nutritious food, unemployment, unhealthy working conditions, unstable home and family life, inadequate education, and living in deprived environments are all associated with poorer health. Lack of access to quality health care and inability to afford pain treatments like psychotherapy, biofeedback, medical procedures, and medications are major barriers to effective care.

Flexing Your Social Muscle

If you've been stuck inside, particularly if you've been home alone for extended periods, your "social muscle" may have atrophied. This isn't an actual muscle, of course, but like all skills, social skills must be used regularly to remain strong and functional. Without regular social contact, conversation, and real-life interaction, your social muscle can wither and weaken. For example, have you ever noticed that the longer you're inside, isolated, playing videogames and watching TV, the harder it can be to step outside into the fray and chaos of life? Socializing, going to the grocery store, and even getting dressed can suddenly feel overwhelming and anxiety-provoking. One way to overcome this hurdle is to slowly, gradually resume social behavior. Pick one small, low-anxiety social interaction that feels safe, like going to the market to buy milk or walking the dog. Then give yourself a new small challenge tomorrow, like saying hello to the cashier. You can also exercise your social muscle virtually by scheduling video dates with far away friends and family, attending virtual interactive classes and workshops, or even participating in online religious communities and gatherings. *Much like pacing for exercise, it's equally as important to pace for social interaction.*

When you're sick or in pain, social support is more important than ever. Tap into your trusted support system—family, friends, teams, religious groups—and spend time with people who care about you. If you don't have a ready-made support group, find some activities that reduce isolation. Here's what Sohita did:

Sohita's Social Medicine

Sohita had neurofibromatosis, a painful genetic condition that caused tumors to grow all over her body and disfigured her face. She was ashamed of her appearance and loathed leaving the house. When she did go outside, she imagined that people looked at her with disgust and ridiculed her appearance. She wore oversized clothes, coats even on the hottest days, and wore a mask even when she didn't need to. She felt lonely, isolated, and alone. Sohita had never been particularly religious, but when she was a child, her family had belonged to a church. Her aunt convinced her to reach out to her local parish to see if they hosted any events. She discovered a monthly book group, and decided to go. When she got out of the car in the church parking lot, nobody stared. When she walked into the building, nobody pointed or ran out. When she introduced herself to the book club, people nodded and smiled. She was so pleased and surprised that she plucked up the courage to speak to the man sitting next to her, Tom. At the end of the evening, Sohita and Tom signed up for monthly book groups together. This reminded her that neurofibromatosis didn't control her, and it didn't define her life. Feeling more confident, she reached out to old friends and organized a game night at her house. It was empowering to explain her condition, get support, and feel accepted. Social interaction helped her feel…normal!

Fuzz Therapy

Social medicine can also come in fuzzy form. Research suggests that having a pet can be good for you: pets can provide comfort, support, and even health benefits. "Fuzz therapy" can decrease levels of cortisol (a stress hormone), lower blood pressure and cholesterol, boost mood, increase feelings of support, ameliorate anxiety, make you laugh and smile, reduce depression and loneliness, improve heart health, and increase feelings of overall well-being.

Petting and cuddling with pets also trigger the release of *oxytocin*—a hormone that induces feelings of connection, bonding, and attachment. In animal studies, oxytocin has been shown to increase pain tolerance and even serve as an anti-inflammatory agent. Furthermore, when an animal relies on you for survival, it can increase your sense of purpose and meaning. Pets can also be motivators: if the dog needs to go out twice a day, this can encourage you to walk more, get more sunlight, and even socialize with other dog owners. No wonder pets often serve as "emotional support animals"! There are even animal-assisted therapy programs in which animals are trained to help rehabilitate patients with acute or chronic diseases.

Your Social Medicine Plan
(circle any that might work!)

How can you increase social support?

- Text or call a friend.

- Find an online support group for others with your same condition.

- Go to the local dog park and befriend dogs and their owners.

- Invite a friend over to watch a comedy or watch the same movie together online even if you're in different places.

- Read in a café.

- Schedule virtual coffee dates with friends around the globe.

- Volunteer at a hospital.

- Visit a local animal shelter and cuddle the cats.

- Sign up for pie-baking classes or virtual cooking lessons with some friends.

- Make a list of books you've been meaning to read and start a book club.

- Join a choir (even if you can't sing!).

- Attend a local or online chronic-pain support group or mindfulness class.

- Sit on your front stoop and talk to a neighbor.

- Attend readings by authors at your local bookstore.

- Join a naturalist or birding group.

- Ask your doctor to connect you with other people with your condition, or to help you start a group/listserv.

- Get the band back together.

- Attend an Alcoholics Anonymous, Narcotics Anonymous, Al-Anon, or other 12-step group.

- Host a weekly card game.

- Join a gym and take a (swimming, yoga, Pilates) class.

- Get a group together to go to the movies.

- Take an art workshop or computer class at a continuing education school.

- Attend a speaker series at a local university.

- Offer to cat-sit friends' cats.

- Ask the barista at the café how her day is going.

- Volunteer at your local library.

- Join a "meetup" group for people who share similar hobbies (for example: bar trivia, British baking shows, dirt biking)

Your ideas:

_____

_____

_____

_____

When Relationships Hurt

While relationships are important, they aren't always healthy. There's a particularly high correlation between unhealthy family systems and chronic pain. In fact, early childhood trauma and family dysfunction—including issues like abuse, domestic violence, physical and verbal conflict, parental mental illness, substance abuse, and ostracization—are significant risk factors for the development and maintenance of chronic pain and other health conditions. Toxic relationships aren't restricted to families: romantic relationships, professional relationships, and friendships can all be unhealthy.

Social interactions can even be *painful*. Think about how you felt, both physically and emotionally, after a breakup, a terrible fight with a parent or spouse, or when you were excluded from something. Did your heart hurt? Did you feel nauseated, or did your body feel heavy or achy? Studies indicate that being socially rejected triggers the same neural circuits that process pain. In fact, "social pain" and "physical pain" are processed by overlapping brain pathways. Love *can* actually hurt! It's therefore important to set boundaries on toxic relationships.

Are there any unhealthy relationships in your life? How do they affect you physically and emotionally?

_____

_____

_____

_____

List two ways you can limit your exposure to toxic relationships:

1. _____

2. _____

How can you set healthy boundaries this week? (*for example: say "no" to plans*)

_____

_____

There is also such a thing as *too much* support. Families can inadvertently contribute to catastrophizing, fear of movement, and unhealthy coping. If someone in your life is doing everything for you—drawing your bath, retrieving food from the fridge, scheduling all of your appointments—this can inadvertently communicate to your brain that you are powerless, disabled, incapable, and incompetent.

Take power back by engaging in activities that allow you to feel competent and confident in the face of pain. This means increasing assurance in your ability to move, use your body, and take care of yourself. Of course, this doesn't apply to everyone all the time, and it doesn't mean that your family and friends shouldn't help you when you need it. They should! It's important to ask for assistance when you need it—no shame in that game. However, an important part of resuming functioning and lowering your pain alarm is teaching your brain that you are capable and powerful, *even if* you have pain. For example, making a meal is the only way to prove to your brain that you *still can.*

List two activities that someone currently does for you that you'd be willing to try to take charge of yourself:

1. _____

2. _____

Managing Fatigue: Drain and Gain

Fatigue and lethargy commonly co-occur with chronic pain. It's therefore important to track your energy, noticing relationships and activities that are draining and those that are energizing. This activity will help you track "drains" and "gains" as you go about your week. Your task in the coming days is to notice times your energy increases—you feel revitalized, invigorated, and more motivated—and times your energy drains, and you feel more lethargic, weak, and fatigued. List your observations in the table below. Then set your intention to reduce one "drain" and increase one "gain" each week. Conserve your energy for healing activities and interactions, and limit the ones that drain you.

Cory's Drains and Gains

DRAIN	GAIN
Fielding emails from my sister and her husband	Writing by the lake
Vacuuming	A trip to the botanical gardens
My colleague Rebecca	Spending time with my cousins
Grocery shopping	Preparing a nice meal

This Week's Goals

Reduce 1 drain: Spend less time with Rebecca.

Increase 1 gain: Set aside 2 hours on Sunday to write by the lake.

Your Drains and Gains

DRAIN	GAIN

This Week's Goals

Reduce 1 drain: _____

Increase 1 gain: _____

Conclusion

You're almost there! Now that you're armed with techniques to improve sleep, exercise, nutrition, fatigue, and social functioning, we'll combine the different parts of this book to help you integrate these strategies into your life. You'll learn how to create a Pain Plan and implement daily structure. This will help you stay motivated, organized, and on track. You've got this!

CHAPTER 8

Putting It All Together

We get better at the things we practice. For example, to get strong arms, lift weights at the gym every day and soon you'll develop muscular biceps. If you want to be a skilled chef, practice cooking and experimenting with recipes every day. When you practice something, the brain pathways dedicated to that skill get bigger and stronger—because neurons that fire together, wire together. This *learning* is the reason why the skills we practice become easier and more automatic.

To break the chronic-pain cycle, rewire your pain system by establishing a *home-practice routine* using pain-management skills—Every. Single. Day. To do this, pick a time and place to practice these skills, even if it's just for ten minutes. It can take a while to establish a new routine, but once you're in the habit of practicing daily, it's easier to keep it up. The most important time to practice is *when pain is medium, low, or absent*—that way, when you have an intense flare-up, your skills will be learned and automatic, and you'll be able to quickly and effectively tackle pain.

Victor's home-practice plan.

Skill: Mindfulness

Daily practice time: 8 p.m. (after dinner, before Netflix)

Practice location: On the couch in the den

How you'll remember: Set phone alarm, practice with Marie-Helene

Your home-practice plan:

Skill: _____

Daily practice time: _____

Practice location: _____

How you'll remember: _____

Five-Things Plan

You now have a boatload of strategies to improve your health by changing triggers, thoughts, emotions, coping strategies, activities, sleep habits, nutrition, and social factors. One great way to put this all together is to create a *Five-Things Plan*. Starting today, your mission is to do five things every day to help yourself feel better. Your five things can include any pain coping skill or activity that lowers pain volume and helps you get your life back. Here's a guideline for choosing daily activities: (1) make sure that one activity is *outdoors*, increasing your exposure to sunlight, people, and serotonin, and (2) make sure that one activity is *physical*, desensitizing brain and body, and promoting the release of serotonin, dopamine, and endorphins. You can combine these two guidelines by moving or exercising outside. If you're trying to get back to work or improve cognitive functioning, make sure to pick at least one brain-based activity like writing or reading to exercise your mind.

Step 1: Make your own personalized Five-Things Menu. Using the strategies in this book combined with personal goals, make your own menu of daily pain-relief skills. For each skill, you can include multiple options for practicing that strategy, as seen on Jessa's menu below. It's fine if some activities fit into two categories; for example, if bike-riding counts as pacing and as a pleasurable activity, you can list it as an option in both categories. Make sure to specify the amount of time you plan to engage in each activity to ensure goals are specific, realistic, and achievable. See Jessa's Five-Things Plan, and then craft your own.

Jessa's Five-Things Menu

Skill	Options
Triggers and emotions	Track & change triggers, teakettle, complete pain recipe worksheet.
Activity pacing	Complete pacing worksheet, knit for 10 minutes, garden for 7 minutes, vacuum for 3 minutes.
Exercise	Walk around the block, ride stationary bike for 20 minutes, 15 push-ups, 10 sit-ups, lift light weights for 3 minutes.
Pacing for work	Go to work for half a day, read a fun book before bed for 20 minutes, 15 minutes of writing.

Distraction	Complete distraction worksheet, visit kittens at local shelter, return book to library, watch movies, draw.
Pleasurable activity	Dance for 10 minutes, garden for 15 minutes, play catch with the dog for 20 minutes, paint with watercolors, ride bike for 20 minutes.
Biofeedback	Hand warming, biofeedback apps.
Relaxation, mindfulness	Mindfulness app, belly breathing, body scan, yoga, Five-Senses Mindfulness.
Imagery	Safe place imagery (imagine a beach), self-healing imagery.
Catch and check thoughts	Tracking Pain Voice, thinking traps, Detective Questions, What Ifs.
Change thoughts	Wise Voice, coping thoughts, Gratitudes and Good Things, gray thoughts, imagine a miracle.
Sleep hygiene	Bed at 11 p.m. and wake at 7 a.m. daily, cover clocks, get out of bed after 20 minutes if anxious or not asleep.
Nutrition	Eat one fruit or vegetable with each meal, replace cookies with nuts for snack.
Social medicine	Invite friends over for game night Friday, swim with Sophia this weekend, call Grandma Ping.
Manage fatigue	Track "drains" and "gains," increase one gain and decrease one drain.

Remember: you don't have to do *all* of the activities in the "options" column—these are just menu items for you to choose from. You can download a blank copy of this menu at http://www .newharbinger.com/46448.

Your Five-Things Menu

Skill	Options
Triggers and emotions	
Activity pacing	
Exercise	
Pacing for work	
Distraction	
Pleasurable activity	
Biofeedback	
Relaxation, mindfulness	
Imagery	
Catch and check thoughts	

Skill	Options
Change thoughts	
Sleep hygiene	
Nutrition	
Social medicine	
Manage fatigue	
Other ideas	1. 2. 3.

Step 2: Establish a reward plan. Rewards help motivate us and can make hard work more fun. If it sounds juvenile to establish a reward system for yourself, consider this: We work for rewards *all the time*. We work to earn money (reward), and eat healthy meals so that we can dig into that pint of ice cream (reward). Summer vacation is a reward, and so is that kiss from your daughter!

Every time you practice five healthy coping skills a day, commit to giving yourself a reward. Your family, spouse, or friends can participate and reward you, or you can treat yourself. Brainstorm rewards you'd like to earn, from small to large, and make a "reward menu" that looks like a birthday wish list. You can earn a small daily reward for doing five things (like a favorite TV show), or add up points after seven successful days to earn a larger reward at the end of the week (a trip, cowboy boots).

Make sure to select rewards you'll actually work for; otherwise, this plan won't be effective. If you notice that the reward isn't motivating enough to get you off the couch and out the door, *it's the wrong reward*. Go back to the drawing board and think of something that'll actually get you going!

Example: Jessa's reward menu:

    Watch 2 episodes of Grey's Anatomy

    New leather boots

    Swim lessons

    Money toward a hot tub

    Trip to Yosemite with the kids

Your reward menu:

_____

_____

_____

_____

_____

Step 3: Select five skills to practice each day this week. Put these skills in the chart below, along with the time and place you'll complete them. Put the chart somewhere visible—your wall, the fridge—as a daily reminder. Commit to using these skills every day for one week. Use the chart below to track daily progress. You can adjust your Five Things the following week or keep the same ones. Make sure that at least one "thing" is exercise and at least one is outdoors. Then select a reward from the reward menu. For this example, Jessa had been wanting to take her children to Yosemite for years. She decided she'd give herself one point daily toward a Yosemite trip, worth a total of seven points. If she did Five Things every day for seven days, she'd earn the trip (1 point × 7 days = 7 points). Remember: rewards are granted only for doing *Five Things each day.* If you earned a reward today, log this in the bottom row. Next week, you can adjust your Five Things or keep the same ones. Jessa's Sunday chart below earned a point:

Jessa's Five Things for <u>Sunday, June 3</u>

Skill	Goal	Completed?
1. Activity pacing	Walk around the block at 9 a.m. for 20 minutes (exercise + outdoors).	Y
2. Relaxation, mindfulness	Mindfulness app: body scan at 9 p.m.	Y
3. Cognitive	Write out Wise Voice coping thoughts at noon.	Y
4. Nutrition	Eat one fruit or vegetable with each meal: grapes with breakfast, apple with lunch, salad with dinner.	Y
5. Social connection	Invite a friend over for Friday game night.	Y
Reward: 1 point toward Yosemite trip!		

You can download a blank copy of this chart at http://www.newharbinger.com/46448.

Your Five Things for (date) _____

Skill	Goal	Completed?
1.		
2.		
3.		
4.		
5.		
Reward:		

Step 4. Track weekly progress. Use the table below to track weekly progress and rewards. For example, after one week, Jessa is close to earning her Yosemite trip, but isn't quite there because she used coping strategies only four days out of seven.

Example: Jessa's Weekly Tracker

	Five Things Completed? (Y/N)	Reward (points or items)
Mon.	Y	1 point
Tues.	N	—
Wed.	Y	1 point
Thurs.	Y	1 point
Fri.	N	—
Sat.	N	—
Sun.	Y	1 point
Total	4 days	4 points
Reward?	N	(Almost there!)

Your Weekly Tracker

	Five Things Completed? (Y/N)	Reward (points or items)
Mon.		
Tues.		
Wed.		
Thurs.		
Fri.		
Sat.		
Sun.		
Total		
Reward?		

You can download a blank Weekly Tracker at http://www.newharbinger.com/46448.

Make a Pain Plan

When you feel calm and confident in the face of pain, a flare-up is much less scary. One way to feel prepared is to create a *Pain Plan* for acute flares. A Pain Plan is your plan for a tough day that includes effective coping strategies that work for you. This will give you, your family, and your treatment team a road map for how to handle a tough day. Make a plan for home and one for work.

You can write out your Pain Plan with markers and colorful pens. Tape it to your fridge, put it in your briefcase, give your loved ones a copy, and give one to your physician. This way, if you start feeling bad, everyone will calmly and confidently know exactly what to do—especially *you*. Eli's pain plan for the onset of a migraine looks like this:

Eli's Pain Plan

Home	Work
1. Hydrate, eat something.	1. Hydrate, eat a granola bar.
2. Lie on the couch for 20 minutes.	2. Relax in the conference room for 20 minutes.
3. Cold pack on head.	3. Cold pack on head.
4. Listen to guided workbook audio, use mindfulness apps, belly breathe, body scan.	4. Bring headphones to work to listen to mindfulness apps, belly breathe, body scan.
5. Stretch, go for a walk outside, get fresh air.	5. Stretch in the break room, go for a walk outside, get fresh air.
6. Distract: play with the dog, finish puzzle, BBQ ribs on the grill.	6. Distract: listen to 20 minutes of a podcast, bring Sudoku to work.
7. Self-talk: "I've had 200 migraines this year alone. I can get through this one. This won't last forever."	7. Self-talk: "I've had 200 migraines this year alone. I can get through this one. This won't last forever."
8. Take meds as needed.	8. Take meds as needed.
9. Call a friend for support.	9. Leave the office for 10 minutes and call a friend for support.
10. Schedule 3 coping breaks today; set timer on phone.	10. Schedule 3 work breaks to use coping strategies throughout the day; set timer on phone.

You can download a blank Pain Plan at http://www.newharbinger.com/46448.

Your Pain Plan

Home	Work
1.	1.
2.	2.
3.	3.
4.	4.
5.	5.
6.	6.
7.	7.
8.	8.
9.	9.
10.	10.

You can also create a weekly *Biopsychosocial Pain Plan* for longterm pain management, selecting a few biological, psychological, and social pain-management strategies to make sure that you target all three domains over the course of your week—whether you have a flare or not. Check out Lili's plan to help manage her sickle cell anemia; then create your own. Download a blank Biopsychosocial Pain Plan for next week at http://www.newharbinger.com/46448.

Lili's Biopsychocoial Pain Plan

Biological

1. Get blood transfusion.

2. Pace and exercise (jog or bike) for 20 minutes three times this week.

3. Take medications as prescribed.

4. Hydrate, eat fruits and vegetables with every meal, and take daily vitamin.

5. Practice sleep hygiene.

Psychological

1. Protect one hour of daily relaxation time at noon.

2. Write out negative thoughts about pain and challenge them.

3. See CBT therapist weekly.

4. Self-soothe daily: morning mindfulness practice, calming music, relaxation apps.

5. Teakettle: journal twice this week.

Social

1. Make social plans with friends Tuesday and Saturday nights.

2. Host video chat with online sickle cell support group.

3. Plan weekend hike with kids.

4. Volunteer at the animal shelter twice this month to connect with community.

5. Schedule a girls' movie night.

Your Biopsychosocial Pain Plan

Biological

1. _____

2. _____

3. _____

4. _____

5. _____

Psychological

1. _____

2. _____

3. _____

4. _____

5. _____

Social

1. _____

2. _____

3. _____

4. _____

5. _____

What to Do If You Can't Get Out of Bed

Sometimes pain and illness make us feel stuck: stuck in bed, stuck at home, just stuck. It's too painful to get up, let alone to go outside or work. To overcome this hurdle, try the Five-Step Bed Plan.

Step 1. Think about getting out of bed. Use *imagery*. Visualize yourself successfully standing up and walking around the room. Imagine the feeling of your feet on the floor.

Belly breathe: Take three slow, deep *belly breaths*.

Use self-talk. Notice *Pain Voice*. Listen for *thinking traps*. Talk back and write out why they're not true. Tune in to *Wise Voice* and use *hurt versus harm*: "I've gotten out of bed a million times before. Standing up and moving will not harm my body. Moving is the first step toward helping my pain."

Step 2. Move: Sit up. Get blood flowing to your legs by tensing and releasing your calf and thigh muscles. Press your legs and heels into the mattress, then squeeze them together. "Bicycle" your legs in the air while lying on your back.

Self-talk: "This is just my sensitive pain system giving me a false alarm. Moving hurts, but it won't harm me."

Think of a *reward* you'll give yourself for getting out of bed: eat a delicious meal, watch a show, buy yourself that pizza oven you've wanted. This is hard work, and motivation can help.

Step 3. Hang your legs over the side of the bed. Let your feet touch the floor. Notice how you feel (nervous? frustrated? overwhelmed?) and what's happening in your head. What are you thinking?

Self-talk: Use encouraging, motivating *coping statements*: "I can do this! Just one small step at a time. Pain has been in control for too long. I'm taking my power back."

Belly breathe: Take three slow, deep *belly breaths*.

Step 4. Stand up slowly. Hold on to something if you feel unsteady. Walk toward your reward! Scratch the cat, put money in the jar, jump online, and buy that thing you've been wanting. If you're tracking *Five Things*, make "get out of bed" a thing and give yourself points.

Step 5. Feel proud of yourself for fighting back against Pain Voice, who tells you "you can't." *You can!*

Living a Life You Love

While a combination of pacing, activity-scheduling, sleep hygiene, thought-challenging, mindfulness, relaxation, distraction, and other CBT techniques can be very helpful, there's no instant or magic cure for chronic pain. Even after completing this workbook, you might continue to have some pain. What then?

A critical part of this program is understanding that *you can still live a life you love even if you have some pain.* In fact, this journey is all about figuring out how to do exactly that. By all means, strive to heal, lower pain volume, and improve functioning. But if pain persists, use the strategies in this book to craft a life you love even if you continue to have some discomfort. Add more pleasure, sunshine, activities, nature, friendships, movement, and joy to your life. Given what you've been through, you deserve that! And no one should ever tell you otherwise. If you've been stuck inside without hope, the time to make a change is now. This is the only life you've got—try to make every day one you value.

Navigating Hospital Stays

Medical procedures and hospital stays are common for people living with pain. These can be harrowing and disempowering, and can trigger medical trauma. The more stressed, scared, and powerless you feel, the more pain amplifies and the worse your immune system functions. It's therefore important to brainstorm strategies for feeling safe and soothed in medical settings, so that you have some control.

To best navigate overnight hospital stays and lengthy procedures, consider bringing items that distract and soothe you along with *comfort objects*—any comforting object that reminds you of home, a safe place, or someone you love. This could be your grandfather's watch, a string your daughter ties around your wrist, or a photo of your dog. Read the list of suggestions below, and then make your own personalized list.

SUGGESTED HOSPITAL LIST

Headphones and audio player: music, podcasts, audiobooks

iPad or laptop: movies, TV shows, YouTube

Favorite pillow

Blanket (consider getting a weighted blanket for extra calming comfort)

Books, magazines, e-readers

Slippers, fuzzy socks

Photos (on your phone or printed)

Journal

Favorite cozy clothes

A deck of cards, knitting, or other activities to keep your hands busy

Letters from people you love, including any children in your life

YOUR HOSPITAL LIST

_____

_____

_____

_____

_____

_____

_____

_____

_____

_____

Pain Identity: Who Are You, Really?

It's easy for life to revolve around pain and illness. Indeed, pain wants to consume your entire identity. Pain is the reason you don't see friends, spend less time enjoying family activities, stop playing sports, miss work, and lose touch with your community. It's the thing you think about most, the task demanding so much of your brain space and energy. Pain can take charge of everything—including who you are. As one client said: "I'm the person who spends weekends in the hospital, who's constantly trying new meds, who has to leave work early for doctor's appointments. I'm the person who's always sick and can't go to parties or travel. Pain has overtaken every aspect of my life. *I am my illness.*"

But now that you've read this book, you know that pain isn't in charge—*you are*. Pain no longer gets to dominate your identity or define who you are. You're so much more than your pain! It's time to take your power back. Let's brainstorm what really defines you, who you *actually* are underneath that pain.

MY IDENTITY:

What I like best about myself:

_____

_____

My hobbies:

_____

_____

Subjects I most like to learn about:

_____

_____

Three things I love most in the entire world:

_____

_____

_____

Favorite movies:

_____

_____

Favorite books:

_____

_____

Favorite foods:

_____

_____

People I feel most like myself around:

_____

_____

Three things that make me laugh:

1. _____

2. _____

3. _____

I'm really good at:

_____

_____

My favorite memory:

_____

_____

I'm an interesting person because:

_____

_____

Things in my life I've accomplished that I'm proud of (_winning an art award, drawing a children's book for my nephews, being the kind of person who helps people_):

_____

_____

You are so much more than your pain!

The Beginning

I bet you thought this was going to say "Conclusion." Well, guess what? You've arrived at the beginning. True, it's the end of this workbook—congratulations, you're officially one step closer to a less stressful, less painful life! You hung in there, you did the work, and that requires incredible persistence and determination. But though this book may be ending..._the rest of your life is just beginning._ You've been through so much. You've tried so many treatments. You now carry these pain-management strategies with you wherever you go. Take them out into the world and use them so that _you_ are in charge of your pain!

Acknowledgments

Profound gratitude for Drs. Adriaan Louw and Lorimer Moseley, international experts and professional pain-explainers, for their generous feedback; Dr. Mark Schumacher, UCSF physician extraordinaire, champion of multidisciplinary care, and supporter of pain psychology, for his insightful foreword; and Dr. Matt McKay for believing in this book—and in me. Special thanks to Dr. Anna Lembke for her brave trailblazing, sage counsel, and support; Drs. Victor Yalom, Erik Peper, and Chris Gilbert for their friendship and consultation; Grant Benson, computer doctor and saver-of-books; and Tesilya Hanauer, Jennifer Holder, Ken Knabb, and the amazing New Harbinger staff for their invaluable input.

Resources

Practicing pain-control techniques is easier when you have support and guidance. Here are some great resources, including mindfulness and relaxation practices, guided imagery, books, apps, websites, and more. Try the exercises and apps and see which work best for you. This list is by no means comprehensive, but it's a great place to start.

Guided Audio

Dr. Zoffness's guided relaxation and mindfulness exercises for this book—http://www.newharbinger
.com/46448

Palouse Mindfulness: a free mindfulness-based stress reduction course (left side under "practices")—
https://palousemindfulness.com

Dr. Dawn Buse: guided relaxations—http://dawnbuse.com/relaxation.htm

UCLA Mindful Awareness Research Center meditations—http://marc.ucla.edu/mindful-meditations

Dr. Bob Stahl's dharma talks and guided mindfulness practices—https://dharmaseed.org/teacher/268/

Dr. Kristen Neff's self-compassion meditations—https://self-compassion.org (under "practices")

Dr. Tara Brach's mindfulness meditations—https://www.tarabrach.com/guided-meditations/

Websites

Psychology Today's pain-management column, "Pain, Explained"—www.psychologytoday.com/us
/blog/pain-explained

Dr. Zoffness's website with pain resources (videos, books, websites, apps)—www.zoffness.com

How to find a biofeedback provider—www.bcia.org (under "find a practitioner")

How to find a CBT-I provider for help with sleep:
www.behavioralsleep.org
www.cbti.directory

RELIEF pain news and education—www.relief.news

Practical Pain Management, pain education and resources—www.practicalpainmanagement.com

MyCarePath, apps and resources—www.mycarepath.ca

Pain Revolution, pain education and resources—www.painrevolution.org

Pain organizations with resources:

American Chronic Pain Association—www.theacpa.org/pain-management-tools/resources/profes
sional-groups/

American Academy of Pain Medicine—https://painmed.org/clinician-resources/pain-education-resources
/organizations-dedicated-to-people-with-pain

Articles (Search for these online using article title and journal.)

"Think Pain Is Purely Medical? Think Again." *Psychology Today.*

"What Changes Pain?" *Psychology Today.*

"Research Uncovers Potential Treatment for Chronic Pain." *Psychology Today.*

"Boyfriend Doesn't Have Ebola. Probably." Hyperbole and a Half. (The funniest-ever version of the
pain scale, in case you need to laugh.)

"The Neuroscience of Pain." *The New Yorker.*

"The Biopsychosocial Approach." *Practical Pain Management.*

"Failed Back Surgery Syndrome." *Practical Pain Management.*

"What is the Neuromatrix Theory of Pain?" *Institute for Chronic Pain.*

"Alternatives to Drugs for Treating Pain." *The New York Times.*

"Why Laughter May Be the Best Pain Medicine." *Scientific American.*

Apps

Stop, Breathe & Think: guided relaxation and meditations, plus an "emotional check-in." Exercises
range from 3 to 15 minutes.

Headspace: guided meditation and relaxation strategies.

Calm: guided meditations and relaxation strategies.

Curable Pain Relief: a pain-management app with info and activities.

Relax Melodies: guided meditations with music and nature sounds. Includes audio for sleep.

Breathe2Relax: teaches diaphragmatic breathing. Change "breath settings" to extend your exhale
and facilitate greater relaxation.

Rain Rain: relaxing soundscapes for soothing, studying, relaxing, and sleeping.

BellyBio Interactive Breathing: a biofeedback app that teaches and monitors belly breathing.

List of pain-related apps: https://paindoctor.com/pain-diary-apps/

Videos (Search for these titles online.)

Tame the Beast: It's Time to Rethink Persistent Pain

Understanding Pain in Less Than Five Minutes, and What to Do About It

The Mysterious Science of Pain (Joshua Pate)

Learning How to Manage Pain During Medical Procedures (Stanford)

Why Things Hurt (TED Talk by Lorimer Moseley)

Podcasts

Pain Reframed

Modern Pain Podcast

Healing Pain Podcast

Pain Science and Sensibility

PAINWeek podcasts: www.painweek.org/media/listen

RELIEF News podcasts: https://relief.news/category/podcasts/

(Note: Beware podcast hosts selling get-fixed-quick schemes, a particular "brand" of pain treatment, gadgets, pills, etc. Unfortunately, there's no magic cure for chronic pain, so don't believe anyone promoting one.)

Books

Butler, David, and Lorimer Moseley. *Explain Pain.*

Carney, Colleen, and Rachel Manber. *Quiet Your Mind and Get to Sleep: Solutions to Insomnia for Those with Depression, Anxiety, or Chronic Pain.*

Dahl, JoAnne, and Tobias Lundgren. *Living Beyond Your Pain: Using Acceptance and Commitment Therapy to Ease Chronic Pain.*

Darnall, Beth. *Less Pain, Fewer Pills: Avoid the Dangers of Prescription Opioids and Gain Control over Chronic Pain.*

Davis, Martha, Elizabeth Robbins Eshelman, and Matthew McKay. *The Relaxation & Stress Reduction Workbook.*

Doidge, Norman. *The Brain That Changes Itself: Stories of Personal Triumph from the Frontiers of Brain Science.*

Kabat-Zinn, Jon. *Full Catastrophe Living: Using the Wisdom of Your Body and Mind to Face Stress, Pain, and Illness.*

Lembke, Anna. *Drug Dealer, MD: How Doctors Were Duped, Patients Got Hooked, and Why It's So Hard to Stop.*

Louw, Adriaan. *Why Do I Hurt?: A Patient Book About the Neuroscience of Pain.*

McKay, Matthew, and Peter Rogers. *The Anger Control Workbook.*

Peper, Erik, Katherine Gibney, and Catherine Holt. *Make Health Happen: Training Yourself to Create Wellness.*

Sarno, John. *The Divided Mind: The Epidemic of Mindbody Disorders.*

Sarno, John. *Healing Back Pain: The Mind-Body Connection.*

Stahl, Bob, and Elisha Goldstein. *A Mindfulness-Based Stress Reduction Workbook.*

Thernstrom, Melanie. *The Pain Chronicals: Cures, Myths, Mysteries, Prayers, Diaries, Brain Scans, Healing, and the Science of Suffering.*

Turk, Dennis, and Frits Winter. *The Pain Survival Guide: How to Reclaim Your Life.*

van der Kolk, Bessel. *The Body Keeps the Score: Brain, Mind, and Body in the Healing of Trauma*

Wall, Patrick. *Pain: The Science of Suffering.*

Williams, Mary Beth, and Soili Poijula. *The PTSD Workbook: Simple, Effective Techniques for Overcoming Traumatic Stress Symptoms.* Third Edition.

Zoffness, Rachel. *The Chronic Pain and Illness Workbook for Teens: CBT and Mindfulness-Based Practices to Turn the Volume Down on Pain.*

References

Chapter 1

Arntz, A., and L. Claassens. 2004. "The Meaning of Pain Influences Its Experienced Intensity." *Pain* 109: 20–25.

Atlas, L., and T. Wager. 2012. "How Expectations Shape Pain." *Neuroscience Letters* 520: 140–148.

Beecher, H. K. 1946. "Pain in Men Wounded in Battle." *Annals of Surgery* 123(1): 96–105.

Beecher, H. K. 1956. "Relationship of Significance of Wound to Pain Experiences." *Journal of the American Medical Association* 161(17): 1609–1613.

Berg, L., C. Hellum, Ø. Gjertsen, G. Neckelmann, L. G. Johnsen, K. Storheim, et al. 2013. "Do More MRI Findings Imply Worse Disability or More Intense Low Back Pain? A Cross-sectional Study of Candidates for Lumbar Disc Prosthesis." *Skeletal Radiology* 42(11): 1593–1602.

Bevers, K., L. Watts, N. Kishino, and R. Gatchel. 2016. "The Biopsychosocial Model of the Assessment, Prevention, and Treatment of Chronic Pain." *U.S. Neurology* 12(2): 98–104.

Brinjikji, W., P. H. Luetmer, B. Comstock, B. W. Bresnahan, L. E. Chen, R. A. Deyo, et al. 2015. "Systematic Literature Review of Imaging Features of Spinal Degeneration in Asymptomatic Populations." *American Journal of Neuroradiology* 36(4): 811–816.

Butler, D. S., and G. L. Moseley. 2013. *Explain Pain, Second Edition.* Adelaide: Noigroup Publications.

Colloca, L., and A. J. Barsky. 2020. "Placebo and Nocebo Effects." *New England Journal of Medicine* 382(6): 554–561.

Darnall, B, D. Carr, and M. Schatman. 2017. "Pain Psychology and the Biopsychosocial Model of Pain Treatment: Ethical Imperatives and Social Responsibility." *Pain Medicine* 18: 1413–1415.

Dimsdale, J. E., and R. Dantzer R. 2007. "A Biological Substrate for Somatoform Disorders: Importance of Pathophysiology." *Psychosomatic Medicine* 69(9): 850–854.

Dowell, D., T. M. Haegerich, and R. Chou. 2016. "CDC Guideline for Prescribing Opioids for Chronic Pain—United States, 2016." *Journal of the American Medical Association* 315(15): 1624–1645.

Edwards, R. R., R. H. Dworkin, M. D. Sullivan, D. C. Turk, and A. D. Wasan. 2016. "The Role of Psychosocial Processes in the Development and Maintenance of Chronic Pain." *The Journal of Pain* 17(9): T70–T92.

Fisher, J. P., D. T. Hassan, and N. O'Connor. 1995. "Minerva." *British Medical Journal* 310: 70.

Gatchel, R. J., and A. M. Maddrey. 2004. "The Biopsychosocial Perspective of Pain." In *Healthcare Psychology Handbook, Volume 2,* edited by J. Raczynski and L. Leviton L. Washington, DC: American Psychological Association Press.

Gatchel, R. J., B. Miller, and L. Lou. 2011. "Failed Back Surgery Syndrome." *Practical Pain Management* 4(3): 20–31.

Graham-Engeland, J. E., S. Song, A. Mathur, D. A. Wagstaff, L. C. Klein, C. Whetzel, and W. T. Ayoub. 2019. "Emotional State Can Affect Inflammatory Responses to Pain Among Rheumatoid Arthritis Patients: Preliminary Findings." *Psychological Reports* 122(6): 2026–2049.

Hebb, D. 1949. *The Organization of Behavior. A Neuropsychological Theory.* New York: Wiley.

Institute of Medicine (US) Committee on Advancing Pain Research, Care, and Education. 2011. *Relieving Pain in America: A Blueprint for Transforming Prevention, Care, Education, and Research.* Washington, DC: National Academies Press.

Krebs, E., A. Gravely, S. Nugent, A. C. Jensen, B. DeRonne, E. S. Goldsmith, et al. 2018. "Effect of Opioid vs. Nonopioid Medications on Pain-Related Function in Patients with Chronic Back Pain or Hip or Knee Osteoarthritis Pain: The SPACE Randomized Clinical Trial." *Journal of the American Medical Association* 319(9): 872–882.

Lapate, R. C., H. Lee, T. V. Salomons, E. M. van Reekum, L. L. Greischar, and R. J. Davidson. 2012. "Amygdalar Function Reflects Common Individual Differences in Emotion and Pain Regulation Success." *J Cogn Neurosci* 24: 148–158.

Louw, A., E. J. Puentedura, K. Zimney, and S. Schmidt 2016. "Know Pain, Know Gain? A Perspective on Pain Neuroscience Education in Physical Therapy." *Journal of Orthopaedic and Sports Physical Therapy* 46(3): 131–134.

Louw, A., K. Zimney, E. J. Puentedura, and I. Diener. 2016. "The Efficacy of Pain Neuroscience Education on Musculoskeletal Pain: A Systematic Review of the Literature." *Physiotherapy Theory and Practice* 32(5): 332–355.

Luo, Y., L. C. Hawkley, L. J. Waite, and J. T. Cacioppo. 2012. "Loneliness, Health, and Mortality in Old Age: A National Longitudinal Study." *Social Science and Medicine* 74(6): 907–914.

Malenbaum, S., F. J. Keefe, A. Williams, R. Ulrich, T. J. Somers. 2008. "Pain in Its Environmental Context: Implications for Designing Environments to Enhance Pain Control." *Pain* 134(3): 241–244.

Martucci, K. T., and S. C. Mackey. 2018. "Neuroimaging of Pain: Human Evidence and Clinical Relevance of Central Nervous System Processes and Modulation." *Anesthesiology: The Journal of the American Society of Anesthesiologists* 128(6): 1241–1254.

Meeus, M., J. Nijs, J. Van Oosterwijck, V. Van Alsenoy, and S. Truijen. 2010. "Pain Physiology Education Improves Pain Beliefs in Patients with Chronic Fatigue Syndrome Compared with Pacing and Self-Management Education: A Double-Blind Randomized Controlled Trial." *Archives of Physical Medicine and Rehabilitation* 91(8): 1153–1159.

Meints, S., and R. Edwards. 2018. "Evaluating Psychosocial Contributions to Chronic Pain Outcomes." *Progress in Neuro-Psychopharmacology and Biological Psychiatry* 87(Pt B): 168–182.

Melzack, R. 1999. "From the Gate to the Neuromatrix." *Pain* 82: S121–S126.

Melzack, R., and P. D. Wall. 1965. "Pain Mechanisms: A New Theory." *Science* 150: 971–979.

Melzack, R., T. J. Coderre, J. Kat, and A. L. Vaccarino. 2001. "Central Neuroplasticity and Pathological Pain." *Annals of the New York Academy of Sciences* 933: 157–174.

Moseley, G.L., and D. S. Butler. 2015. "Fifteen Years of Explaining Pain: The Past, Present, and Future." *The Journal of Pain* 16(9): 807–813.

Moseley, G. L., and H. Flor. 2012. "Targeting Cortical Representations in the Treatment of Chronic Pain: A Review." *Neurorehabilitation and Neural Repair* 26(6): 646–652.

Nahin, R. L. 2015. "Estimates of Pain Prevalence and Severity in Adults: United States, 2012." *Journal of Pain* 16(8): 769–780.

Nahin, R. L., R. Boineau, P. S. Khalsa, B. J. Stussman, W. J. Weber. 2016. "Evidence-Based Evaluation of Complementary Health Approaches for Pain Management in the United States." *Mayo Clinic Proceedings* 91(9): 1292–1306.

Orenius, T. I., T. T. Raij, A. Nuortimo, P. Näätänen, J. Lipsanen, and H. Karlsson. 2017. "The Interaction of Emotion and Pain in the Insula and Secondary Somatosensory Cortex." *Neuroscience* 349: 185–194.

Ossipov, M. H., K. Morimura, and F. Porreca. 2014. "Descending Pain Modulation and Chronification of Pain." *Current Opinion in Supportive and Palliative Care* 8: 143–151.

Tick, H., A. Nielsen, K. R. Pelletier, R. Bonakdar, S. Simmons, R. Glick, et al. 2018. "Evidence-Based Nonpharmacologic Strategies for Comprehensive Pain Care: The Consortium Pain Task Force White Paper." *Explore: The Journal of Science and Healing* 14(3): 177–211.

Chapter 2

Adler-Neal, A. L., N. M. Emerson, S. R. Farris, Y. Jung, R. C. Coghill, and F. Zeidan. 2019. "Brain Moderators Supporting the Relationship Between Depressive Mood and Pain." *Pain* 160(9): 2028–2035

Ahmad, A. H., and R. Zakaria. 2015. "Pain in Times of Stress." *Malaysian Journal of Medical Science* 22(Special Issue): 52–61.

American Psychiatric Association. May 7, 2018. "Americans Say They are More Anxious than a Year Ago; Baby Boomers Report Greatest Increase in Anxiety." Retrieved from: https://www.psychia try.org/newsroom/news-releases/americans-say-they-are-more-anxious-than-a-year-ago-baby -boomers-report-greatest-increase-in-anxiety

Bachhuber, M. A., S. Hennessy, C. O. Cunningham, and J. L. Starrels. 2016. "Increasing Benzodiazepine Prescriptions and Overdose Mortality in the United States, 1996–2013." *American Journal of Public Health* 106(4): 686–688.

Berna, C., S. Leknes, E. A. Holmes, R. R. Edwards, G. M. Goodwin, and I. Tracy. 2010. "Induction of Depressed Mood Disrupts Emotion Regulation Neurocircuitry and Enhances Pain Unpleasantness." *Biological Psychiatry* 67: 1083–1090.

Burns, J. W., W. R. Nielson, M. P. Jensen, A. Heapy, R. Czlapinski, and R. D. Kerns. (2015). "Specific and General Therapeutic Mechanisms in Cognitive Behavioral Treatment of Chronic Pain." *Journal of Consulting and Clinical Psychology* 83(1): 1–11.

Bushnell, M. C., M. Čeko, and L. A. Low. 2013. "Cognitive and Emotional Control of Pain and Its Disruption in Chronic Pain." *Nature Reviews Neuroscience* 14(7): 502–511.

Ernst, M. M., H. L. O'Brien, and S. W. Powers. 2015. "Cognitive-Behavioral Therapy: How Medical Providers Can Increase Patient and Family Openness and Access to Evidence-Based Multimodal Therapy for Pediatric Migraine." *Headache* 55(10): 1382–1396.

Felitti, V. J., R. F. Anda, D. Nordenberg, D. F. Williamson, A. M. Spitz, V. Edwards, et al. 1998. "Relationship of Childhood Abuse and Household Dysfunction to Many of the Leading Causes of Death in Adults." *American Journal of Preventive Medicine* 14(4): 245–258.

Finnerup, N. B. 2019. "Nonnarcotic Methods of Pain Management." *New England Journal of Medicine* 380(25): 2440–2448.

Fishbain, D. A., A. Pulikal, J. E. Lewis, and J. Gao. 2017. "Chronic Pain Types Differ in Their Reported Prevalence of Post-Traumatic Stress Disorder (PTSD) and There Is Consistent Evidence That Chronic Pain Is Associated with PTSD: An Evidence-Based Structured Systematic Review." *Pain Medicine* 18(4): 711–735.

Flor, H. 2014. "Psychological Pain Interventions and Neurophysiology: Implications for a Mechanism-Based Approach." *American Psychologist* 69(2): 188–196.

Garland, E., C. Brintz, A. Hanley, E. Roseen, R. Atchley, S. Gaylord, et al. 2020. "Mind-Body Therapies for Opioid-Treated Pain: A Systematic Review and Meta-analysis." *Journal of the American Medical Association Internal Medicine* 180(1): 91–105.

Gatchel, R., Y. Peng, M. Peters, P. Fuchs, and D. Turk. 2007. "The Biopsychosocial Approach to Chronic Pain: Scientific Advances and Future Directions." *Psychological Bulletin* 133(4): 581–624.

Hofmann, S. G., A. Asnaani, I. J. Vonk, A. T. Sawyer, and A. Fang. 2012. "The Efficacy of Cognitive Behavioral Therapy: A Review of Meta-analyses." *Cognitive Therapy and Research* 36(5): 427–440.

Hughes, K., M. A. Bellis, K. A. Hardcastle, D. Sethi, A. Butchart, C. Mikton, et al. 2017. "The Effect of Multiple Adverse Childhood Experiences on Health: A Systematic Review and Meta-analysis." *The Lancet Public Health* 2(8): e356–e366.

Kerns, R. D., J. Sellinger, and B. R. Goodin. 2011. "Psychological Treatment of Chronic Pain." *Annual Review of Clinical Psychology* 7: 411–434.

Kroenke, K., J. Wu, M. J. Bair, E. E. Krebs, T. M. Damush, and W. Tu. 2011. "Reciprocal Relationship Between Pain and Depression: A 12-Month Longitudinal Analysis in Primary Care." *The Journal of Pain.* 12(9): 964–973.

Lumley, M. A., J. L. Cohen, G. S. Borszcz, A. Cano, A. M. Radcliffe, L. S. Porter, et al. 2011. "Pain and Emotion: A Biopsychosocial Review of Recent Research." *Journal of Clinical Psychology.* 67(9): 942–968.

Majeed, M. H., and D. M. Sudak. 2017. "Cognitive Behavioral Therapy for Chronic Pain—One Therapeutic Approach for the Opioid Epidemic." *Journal of Psychiatric Practice* 23: 409–414.

Malfliet, A., I. Coppieters, P. Van Wilgen, J. Kregel, R. De Pauw, M. Dolphens, et al. 2017. "Brain Changes Associated with Cognitive and Emotional Factors in Chronic Pain: A Systematic Review." *European Journal of Pain* 21(5): 769–786.

Petersen, G. L., N. B. Finnerup, K. Grosen, H. K. Pilegaard, I. Tracey, F. Benedetti, et al. 2014. "Expectations and Positive Emotional Feelings Accompany Reductions in Ongoing and Evoked Neuropathic Pain Following Placebo Interventions." *Pain* 155: 2687–2698.

Rivat, C., C. Becker, A. Blugeot, B. Zeau, A. Mauborgne, M. Pohl, et al. 2010. "Chronic Stress Induces Transient Spinal Neuroinflammation, Triggering Sensory Hypersensitivity and Long-Lasting Anxiety-Induced Hyperalgesia." *Pain* 150: 358–368.

Roy, M., M. Piché, J. I. Chen, I. Peretz, and P. Rainville. 2009. "Cerebral and Spinal Modulation of Pain by Emotions." *Proceedings of the National Academy of Sciences* 106(49): 20900–20905.

Schlereth, T., and F. Birklein. 2008. "The Sympathetic Nervous System and Pain." *Neuromolecular Medicine* 10(3): 141–147.

Skelly, A. C., R. Chou, J. R. Dettori, J. A. Turner, J. L. Friedly, S. D. Rundell, et al. June 2018. "Noninvasive Nonpharmacological Treatment for Chronic Pain: A Systematic Review." *Comparative Effectiveness Review.* AHRQ Publication No. 18-EHC013-EF. Rockville, MD: Agency for Healthcare Research and Quality.

Stellar, J. E., N. John-Henderson, C. L. Anderson, A. M. Gordon, G. D. McNeil, and D. Keltner. 2015. "Positive Affect and Markers of Inflammation: Discrete Positive Emotions Predict Lower Levels of Inflammatory Cytokines." *Emotion* 15: 129–133.

Sturgeon, J. A. 2014. "Psychological Therapies for the Management of Chronic Pain." *Psychology Research and Behavior Management* 7: 115–124.

Tick, H., A. Nielsen, K. R. Pelletier, R. Bonakdar, S. Simmons, R. Glick, et al. 2018. "Evidence-Based Nonpharmacologic Strategies for Comprehensive Pain Care: The Consortium Pain Task Force White Paper." *Explore: The Journal of Science and Healing* 14(3): 177–211.

Williams, A. C., C. Eccleston, and S. Morley. 2012. "Psychological Therapies for the Management of Chronic Pain (Excluding Headache) in Adults." *Cochrane Database Syst Rev.* 11:CD007407.

Yoshino, A., Y. Okamoto, G. Okada, M. Takamura, N. Ichikawa, C. Shibasaki, et al. 2018. "Changes in Resting-State Brain Networks After Cognitive-Behavioral Therapy for Chronic Pain." *Psychological Medicine* 48(7): 1148–1156.

Young, S. N. 2007. "How to Increase Serotonin in the Human Brain Without Drugs." *Journal of Psychiatry and Neuroscience* 32(6): 394–399.

Zhang, J. M., and J. An. 2007. "Cytokines, Inflammation and Pain." *International Anesthesiology Clinics* 45: 27–37.

Chapter 3

Altier, N., and J. Stewart. 1999. "The Role of Dopamine in the Nucleus Accumbens in Analgesia." *Life Sciences* 65: 2269–2287.

Ambrose, K. R., and Y. M. Golightly. 2015. "Physical Exercise as Non-pharmacological Treatment of Chronic Pain: Why and When." *Best Practice & Research. Clinical Rheumatology.* 29(1): 120–130.

Antcliff, D., P. Keeley, M. Campbell, S. Woby, A. M. Keenan, and L. McGowan. 2018. "Activity Pacing: Moving Beyond Taking Breaks and Slowing Down." *Quality of Life Research* 27(7): 1933–1935.

Bantick, S. J., R. G. Wise, A. Ploghaus, S. Clare, S. N. Smith, and I. Tracey. 2002. "Imaging How Attention Modulates Pain in Humans Using Functional MRI." *Brain* 125(2): 310–319.

Birnie, K., C. Chambers, and C. Spellman. 2017. "Mechanisms of Distraction in Acute Pain Perception and Modulation." *Pain* 158: 1012–1013.

Booth, J., G. L. Moseley, M. Schiltenwolf, A. Cashin, M. Davies, and M. Hübscher. 2017. "Exercise for Chronic Musculoskeletal Pain: A Biopsychosocial Approach." *Musculoskeletal Care* 15(4): 413–421.

Graham-Engeland, J. E., S. Song, A. Mathur, D. A. Wagstaff, L. C. Klein, C. Whetzel, et al. 2019. "Emotional State Can Affect Inflammatory Responses to Pain Among Rheumatoid Arthritis Patients: Preliminary Findings." *Psychological Reports* 122(6): 2026–2049.

Hassett, A. L., and D. A. Williams. 2011. "Non-pharmacological Treatment of Chronic Widespread Musculoskeletal Pain." *Best Practice & Research. Clinical Rheumatology* 25: 299–309.

Hunt, M. G., R. Marx, C. Lipson, and J. Young. 2018. "No More FOMO: Limiting Social Media Decreases Loneliness and Depression." *Journal of Social and Clinical Psychology* 37(10): 751–768.

Linehan, M. 2014. *DBT Skills Training Manual.* New York: Guilford Publications.

Luque-Suarez, A., J. Martinez-Calderon, and D. Falla. 2019. "Role of Kinesiophobia on Pain, Disability and Quality of Life in People Suffering from Chronic Musculoskeletal Pain: A Systematic Review." *British Journal of Sports Medicine* 53: 554–559.

Martin, M. Y., L. A. Bradley, R. W. Alexander, G. S. Alarcón, M. Triana-Alexander, L. A. Aaron, et al. 1996. "Coping Strategies Predict Disability in Patients with Primary Fibromyalgia." *Pain* 68: 45–53.

Melzack, R., and P. D. Wall. 1965. "Pain Mechanisms: A New Theory." *Science* 150: 971–979.

Murphy, J., J. McKellar, S. Raffa, M. Clark, R. Kerns, and B. Karlin. 2014. *Cognitive Behavioral Therapy for Chronic Pain Among Veterans: Therapist Manual.* Washington, DC: U.S. Department of Veterans Affairs.

Torta, D. M., V. Legrain, A. Mouraux, and E. Valentini. 2017. "Attention to Pain! A Neurocognitive Perspective on Attentional Modulation of Pain in Neuroimaging Studies." *Cortex* 89: 120–134.

Villemure, C., and M. C. Bushnell. 2009. "Mood Influences Supraspinal Pain Processing Separately from Attention." *Journal of Neuroscience* 29(3): 705–715.

Chapter 4

American Migraine Foundation. Nov 12, 2016. "Biofeedback and Relaxation Training for Headaches." Retrieved from: https://americanmigrainefoundation.org/resource-library/biofeedback-and-relaxation-training-for-headaches/

Andrasik, F. 2010. "Biofeedback in Headache: An Overview of Approaches and Evidence." *Cleveland Clinic Journal of Medicine* 77(Suppl 3): S72–S76.

Bear, M. F., B. W. Connors, and M. A. Paradiso (Eds.). 2007. *Neuroscience: Exploring the Brain (Ed. 2)*. Philadelphia, PA: Lippincott Williams & Wilkins.

Davidson, R. J., J. Kabat-Zinn, J. Schumacher, M. Rosenkranz, D. Muller, S. F. Santorelli, et al. 2003. "Alterations in Brain and Immune Function Produced by Mindfulness Meditation." *Psychosomatic Medicine* 65(4): 564–570.

Fjorback, L. O., M. Arendt, E. Ornbøl, P. Fink, and H. Walach. 2011. "Mindfulness-Based Stress Reduction and Mindfulness-Based Cognitive Therapy: A Systematic Review of Randomized Controlled Trials." *Acta Psychiatrica Scandinavica* 124(2): 102–119.

Franke, H. A. 2014. "Toxic Stress: Effects, Prevention and Treatment." *Children* (Basel, Switzerland) 1(3): 390–402.

Garland, E., C. Brintz, A. Hanley, E. Roseen, R. Atchley, S. Gaylord, et al. 2020. "Mind-Body Therapies for Opioid-Treated Pain: A Systematic Review and Meta-analysis." *Journal of the American Medical Association Internal Medicine* 180(1): 91–105.

Gatchel, R. J., R. C. Robinson, C. Pulliam, and A. M. Maddrey. 2003. "Biofeedback with Pain Patients: Evidence for Its Effectiveness." *Seminars in Pain Medicine* 1(2): 55–66.

Hilton, L., S. Hempel, B. A. Ewing, E. Apaydin, L. Xenakis, S. Newberry, et al. 2017. "Mindfulness Meditation for Chronic Pain: Systematic Review and Meta-analysis." *Annals of Behavioral Medicine* 51(2): 199–213.

Martucci, K. T., and S. C. Mackey. 2018. "Neuroimaging of Pain: Human Evidence and Clinical Relevance of Central Nervous System Processes and Modulation." *Anesthesiology: The Journal of the American Society of Anesthesiologists* 128(6): 1241–1254.

Moseley, G. L., N. Zalucki, F. Birklein, J. Marinus, J. J. van Hilten, and H. Luomajoki. 2008. "Thinking About Movement Hurts: The Effect of Motor Imagery on Pain and Swelling in People with Chronic Arm Pain." *Arthritis Care and Research* 59: 623–631.

Peper, E., and K. H. Gibney. 2003. "A Teaching Strategy for Successful Hand Warming." *Somatics* 14: 26–30.

Zeidan, F., K. T. Martucci, R. A. Kraft, N. S. Gordon, J. G. McHaffie, and R. C. Coghill. 2011. "Brain Mechanisms Supporting the Modulation of Pain by Mindfulness Meditation." *Journal of Neuroscience* 31(14): 5540–5548.

Zeidan, F., J. N. Baumgartner, and R. C. Coghill. 2019. "The Neural Mechanisms of Mindfulness-Based Pain Relief: A Functional Magnetic Resonance Imaging-Based Review and Primer." *Pain Reports* 4(4): e759.

Chapter 5

Arntz, A., and L. Claassens. 2004. "The Meaning of Pain Influences Its Experienced Intensity." *Pain* 109: 20–25.

Atlas, L., and T. Wager. 2012. "How Expectations Shape Pain." *Neuroscience Letters* 520: 140–148.

Bannister, K., and A. H. Dickenson. 2016. "What Do Monoamines Do in Pain Modulation?" *Current Opinion in Supportive and Palliative Care* 10: 143–148.

Bushnell, M. C., M. Čeko, and L. A. Low. 2013. "Cognitive and Emotional Control of Pain and Its Disruption in Chronic Pain." *Nature Reviews Neuroscience* 14(7): 502–511.

Cano-García, F. J., L. Rodríguez-Franco, and A. M. López-Jiménez. 2013. "Locus of Control Patterns in Headaches and Chronic Pain." *Pain Research & Management* 18(4): e48–e54.

Colloça, L., and A. J. Barsky. 2020. "Placebo and Nocebo Effects." *New England Journal of Medicine* 382(6): 554–561.

Eklund, A., D. De Carvalho, I. Pagé, A. Wong, M. S. Johansson, K. A. Pohlman, et al. 2019. "Expectations Influence Treatment Outcomes in Patients with Low Back Pain. A Secondary Analysis of Data from a Randomized Clinical Trial." *European Journal of Pain* 23(7): 1378–1389.

Keedy, N. H., V. J. Keffala, E. M. Altmaier, and J. J. Chen. 2014. "Health Locus of Control and Self-Efficacy Predict Back Pain Rehabilitation Outcomes." *Iowa Orthopedic Journal* 34: 158–165.

Kiecolt-Glaser, J. K., L. McGuire, T. F. Robles, and R. Glaser. 2002. "Psychoneuroimmunology: Psychological Influences on Immune Function and Health." *Journal of Consulting and Clinical Psychology* 70(3): 537–547.

Racine, M. 2018. "Chronic Pain and Suicide Risk: A Comprehensive Review." *Progress in Neuro-Psychopharmacology and Biological Psychiatry* 87(Pt B): 269–280.

Stellar, J. E., N. John-Henderson, C. L. Anderson, A. M. Gordon, G. D. McNeil, and D. Keltner. 2015. "Positive Affect and Markers of Inflammation: Discrete Positive Emotions Predict Lower Levels of Inflammatory Cytokines." *Emotion* 15: 129–133.

Sullivan, M. J. L., S. R. Bishop, and J. Pivik. 1995. "The Pain Catastrophizing Scale: Development and Validation." *Psychological Assessment* 7: 524–532.

Tinnermann, A., S. Geuter, C. Sprenger, J. Finsterbusch, and C. Büchel. 2017. "Interactions Between Brain and Spinal Cord Mediate Value Effects in Nocebo Hyperalgesia." *Science* 358: 105–108.

Wiech, K. 2016. "Deconstructing the Sensation of Pain: The Influence of Cognitive Processes on Pain Perception." *Science* 354(6312): 584–587.

Zhang, J. M., and J. An. 2007. "Cytokines, Inflammation and Pain." *International Anesthesiology Clinics* 45: 27–37.

Chapter 6

Bedell, S. E., T. B. Graboys, E. Bedell, and B. Lown. 2004. "Words That Harm, Words That Heal." *Archives of Internal Medicine* 164: 1365–1368.

Dunne, S., D. Sheffield, and J. Chilcot. 2018. "Brief Report: Self-Compassion, Physical Health, and the Mediating Role of Health-Promoting Behaviours." *Journal of Health Psychology* 23: 993–999.

Fox, G. R., J. Kaplan, H. Damasio, and A. Damasio. 2015. "Neural Correlates of Gratitude." *Frontiers in Psychology* 6: 1491.

Grant, A. M., and F. Gino. 2010. "A Little Thanks Goes a Long Way: Explaining Why Gratitude Expressions Motivate Prosocial Behavior." *Journal of Personality and Social Psychology* 98(6): 946–955.

Hassett, A. L. 2018. "Remaining Positive About Positive Psychological Interventions for Pain." *Journal of the American Medical Association Network Open* 1(5): e182531.

Hayter, M. R., and D. S. Dorstyn. 2014. "Resilience, Self-Esteem, and Self-Compassion in Adults with Spina Bifida." *Spinal Cord* 52(2): 167–171.

Hill, P. L., M. Allemand, and B. W. Roberts. 2013. "Examining the Pathways Between Gratitude and Self-Rated Physical Health Across Adulthood." *Personality and Individual Differences* 54: 92–96.

Kini, P., J. Wong, S. McInnis, N. Gabana, and J. W. Brown. 2016. "The Effects of Gratitude Expression on Neural Activity." *NeuroImage* 128: 1–10.

Matthewson, G. M., C. W. Woo, M. C. Reddan, and T. D. Wager. 2019. "Cognitive Self-Regulation Influences Pain-Related Physiology." *Pain* 160(10): 2338–2349.

Natraj, N., and K. Ganguly. 2018. "Shaping Reality Through Mental Rehearsal." *Neuron.* 97(5): 998–1000

Nery-Hurwit, M., J. Yun, and V. Ebbeck. 2018. "Examining the Roles of Self-Compassion and Resilience on Health-Related Quality of Life for Individuals with Multiple Sclerosis." *Disability and Health Journal* 11(2): 256–261.

Palermo, T. M. 2012. Cognitive-Behavioral Therapy for Chronic Pain in Children and Adolescents. New York: Oxford University Press.

Sansone, R. A., and L. A. Sansone. 2010. "Gratitude and Well Being: The Benefits of Appreciation," *Psychiatry (Eldgmont)* 7(11): 18–22.

Chapter 7

Akbari, F., M. Dehghani, A. Khatibi, and T. Vervoort. (2016). "Incorporating Family Function into Chronic Pain Disability: The Role of Catastrophizing." *Pain Research and Management* 2016:2938596.

Ambrose, K. R., and Y. M. Golightly. 2015. "Physical Exercise as Non-pharmacological Treatment of Chronic Pain: Why and When." *Best Practice & Research. Clinical Rheumatology* 29(1): 120–130.

Bannister, K., and A. H. Dickenson. 2016. "What Do Monoamines Do in Pain Modulation?" *Current Opinion in Supportive and Palliative Care* 10: 143–148.

Barile, J. P., V. J. Edwards, S. S. Dhingra, and W. W. Thompson. 2015. "Associations Among County-Level Social Determinants of Health, Child Maltreatment, and Emotional Support on Health-Related Quality of Life in Adulthood." *Psychology of Violence* 5(2): 183–191.

Barton, J., and J. Pretty. 2010. "What Is the Best Dose of Nature and Green Exercise for Improving Mental Health? A Multi-Study Analysis." *Environmental Science and Technology* 44(10): 3947–3955.

Beetz, A., K. Uvnäs-Moberg, H. Julius, and K. Kotrschal. 2012. "Psychosocial and Psychophysiological Effects of Human-Animal Interactions: The Possible Role of Oxytocin." *Frontiers in Psychology* 3: 234.

Booth, F., C. Roberts, and M. Laye. 2012. "Lack of Exercise Is a Major Cause of Chronic Diseases." *Comprehensive Physiology* 2: 1143–1211.

Brasure, M., E. Fuchs, R. MacDonald, V. A. Nelson, E. Koffel, C. M. Olson, et al. 2016. "Psychological and Behavioral Interventions for Managing Insomnia Disorder: An Evidence Report for a Clinical Practice Guideline by the American College of Physicians." *Annals of Internal Medicine* 165: 113–124.

Bratman, G. N., J. P. Hamilton, and G. C. Daily. 2012. "The Impacts of Nature Experience on Human Cognitive Function and Mental Health." *Annals of the New York Academy of Sciences* 1249(1): 118–136.

Cacioppo, J. T., S. Cacioppo, J. P. Capitanio, and S. W. Cole. 2015. "The Neuroendocrinology of Social Isolation." *Annual Review of Psychology* 66: 733–767.

Diette, G. B., N. Lechtzin, E. Haponik, A. Devrotes, and H. R. Rubin. 2003. "Distraction Therapy with Nature Sights and Sounds Reduces Pain During Flexible Bronchoscopy: A Complementary Approach to Routine Analgesia." *Chest* 123: 941–948.

Dölen, G., A. Darvishzadeh, K. W. Huang, and R. C. Malenka. 2013. "Social Reward Requires Coordinated Activity of Nucleus Accumbens Oxytocin and Serotonin." *Nature* 501: 179–184.

Falbe, J., K. K. Davison, R, L. Franckle, C. Ganter, S. L. Gortmaker, L. Smith, et al. 2015. "Sleep Duration, Restfulness, and Screens in the Sleep Environment." *Pediatrics* 135(2): e367–e375.

Felitti, V., R. Anda, D. Nordenberg, D. Williamson, A. Spitz, V. Edwards, et al. 2019. "Relationship of Childhood Abuse and Household Dysfunction to Many of the Leading Causes of Death in Adults: The Adverse Childhood Experiences (ACE) Study." *American Journal of Preventive Medicine* 56(6): 774–786.

Gardner, A. 2014. "Ten Exercises for People in Pain." Retrieved from https://www.health.com/condition/fibromyalgia/10-exercises-for-people-in-pain.

Hartig, T., R. Mitchell, S. De Vries, and H. Frumkin. 2014. "Nature and Health." *Annual Review of Public Health* 35: 207–228.

Holt-Lunstad, J., T. Smith, M. Baker, T. Harris, and D. Stephenson. 2015. "Loneliness and Social Isolation as Risk Factors for Mortality: A Meta-Analytic Review." *Perspectives on Psychological Science* 10: 227–237.

Johnson, M. I. 2019. "The Landscape of Chronic Pain: Broader Perspectives." *Medicina* 55(5): E182.

Karayannis, N., I. Baumann, J. Sturgeon, M. Melloh, and S. Mackey. 2019. "The Impact of Social Isolation on Pain Interference: A Longitudinal Study." *Annals of Behavioral Medicine* 53(1): 65–74.

Koffel, E., S. M. McCurry, M. T. Smith, and M. V. Vitiello. 2019. "Improving Pain and Sleep in Middle-Aged and Older Adults: The Promise of Behavioral Sleep Interventions." *Pain* 160(3): 529–534.

Krach, S., F. M. Paulus, M. Bodden, and T. Kircher. 2010. "The Rewarding Nature of Social Interactions." *Frontiers in Behavioral Neuroscience* 4: 22.

Kross, E., M. Berman., W. Mischel., E. Smith, and T. Wager. 2011. "Social Rejection Shares Somatosensory Representations with Physical Pain." *Proceedings of the National Academy of Sciences* 108(15): 6270–6275.

Luo, Y., L. C. Hawkley, L. J. Waite, and J. T. Cacioppo. 2012. "Loneliness, Health, and Mortality in Old Age: A National Longitudinal Study." *Social Science and Medicine* 74(6): 907–914.

Malenbaum, S., F. J. Keefe, A. Williams, R. Ulrich, and T. J. Somers. 2008. "Pain in Its Environmental Context: Implications for Designing Environments to Enhance Pain Control." *Pain* 134(3): 241–244.

Mayo Clinic. Dec. 15. 2017. "Nutrition and Pain." https://www.mayoclinic.org/nutrition-and-pain/art-20208638.

Mayo Clinic. N.D. "Migraine: Symptoms and Causes." https://www.mayoclinic.org/diseases-conditions/migraine-headache/symptoms-causes/syc-20360201

Mead, M. N. 2008. "Benefits of Sunlight: A Bright Spot for Human Health." *Environmental Health Perspectives* 116(4): A160–A167.

Mubanga, M., L. Byberg, C. Nowak, A. Egenvall, P. K. Magnusson, E. Ingelsson, el al. 2017. "Dog Ownership and the Risk of Cardiovascular Disease and Death—A Nationwide Cohort Study." *Scientific Reports* 7(1): 15821.

Murillo-Garcia, A., S. Villafaina, J. C. Adsuar, N. Gusi, and D. Collado-Mateo. 2018. "Effects of Dance on Pain in Patients with Fibromyalgia: A Systematic Review and Meta-analysis." *Evidence-Based Complementary and Alternative Medicine* 8709748.

National Institutes of Health. "Vitamin D Fact Sheet for Health Professionals." https://ods.od.nih.gov/factsheets/VitaminD-HealthProfessional.

Nijs, J., O. Mairesse, D. Neu, L. Leysen, L. Danneels, B. Cagnie, et al. 2018. "Sleep Disturbances in Chronic Pain: Neurobiology, Assessment, and Treatment in Physical Therapist Practice." *Physical Therapy* 98(5): 325–335.

Palermo, T. M., C. R. Valrie, and C. W. Karlson. 2014. "Family and Parent Influences on Pediatric Chronic Pain: A Developmental Perspective." *American Psychologist* 69(2): 142–152.

Pearce, E., R. Wlodarski, A. Machin, and R. Dunbar. 2017. "Variation in the ß endorphin, Oxytocin, and Dopamine Receptor Genes Is Associated with Different Dimensions of Human Sociality." *Proceedings of the National Academy of Sciences of the United States of America* 114(20): 5300–5305.

Qaseem, A., D. Kansagara, M. A. Forciea, M. Cooke, and T. D. Denberg for the Clinical Guidelines Committee of the American College of Physicians. 2016. "Management of Chronic Insomnia Disorder in Adults: A Clinical Practice Guideline from the American College of Physicians." *Annals of Internal Medicine* 165(2): 125–133.

Sturgeon, J. A., and A. J. Zautra. 2016. "Social Pain and Physical Pain: Shared Paths to Resilience." *Pain Management* 6(1): 63–74.

Tick, H. 2015. "Nutrition and Pain." *Physical Medicine and Rehabilitation Clinics of North America* 26: 309–320.

Trauer. J. M., M. Y. Qian, J. S. Doyle, S. M. Rajaratnam, and D. Cunnington. 2015. "Cognitive Behavioral Therapy for Chronic Insomnia: A Systematic Review and Meta-analysis." *Annals of Internal Medicine* 163: 191–204.

U.S. Department of Health and Human Services (US DHHS, May 9, 2019). "Pain Management Best Practices Inter-Agency Task Force Report: Updates, Gaps, Inconsistencies, and Recommendations." https://www.hhs.gov/ash/advisory-committees/pain/reports/index.html.

Van Hecke, O., N. Torrance, and B. H. Smith. 2013. "Chronic Pain Epidemiology—Where Do Lifestyle Factors Fit In?" *British Journal of Pain* 7: 209–217.

Young, S. N. 2007. "How to Increase Serotonin in the Human Brain Without Drugs." *Journal of Psychiatry and Neuroscience* 32(6): 394–399.

Chapter 8

Harris, S., S. Morley, and S. Barton. 2003. "Role Loss and Emotional Adjustment in Chronic Pain." *Pain* 105: 363–370.

Hebb, D. 1949. *The Organization of Behavior: A Neuropsychological Theory.* New York: Wiley.

Rachel Zoffness, MS, PhD, is faculty at the UCSF School of Medicine, where she teaches pain education for medical residents and interns, and serves on the steering committee of the American Association of Pain Psychology. She is a pain psychologist, author, medical consultant, and educator specializing in chronic pain and illness. She is author of *The Chronic Pain and Illness Workbook for Teens*; piloted the *Psychology Today* column, Pain, Explained; and is a 2020 Mayday Pain Advocacy Fellow. She was trained at Brown University, Columbia University, University of California San Diego, San Diego State University, and Mount Sinai St. Luke's Hospital. She provides lectures and trainings for multidisciplinary health care providers, and serves as a consultant to medical professionals and hospitals around the world.

Foreword writer **Mark A. Schumacher, MD, PhD**, is professor and chief of the division of pain medicine in the department of anesthesia and perioperative care at the University of California, San Francisco (UCSF). Schumacher is director of the UCSF Pain and Addiction Research Center; recently served on the National Academies of Science, Engineering, and Medicine Committee; and coauthored a report on the opioid epidemic. Throughout his career, he has sought ways to communicate the science and practice of pain medicine, including previously directing an NIH Center of Excellence in Pain Education at UCSF.

MORE BOOKS from
NEW HARBINGER PUBLICATIONS

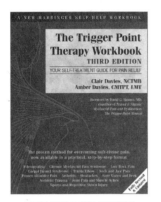
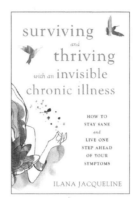
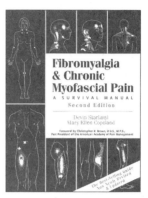
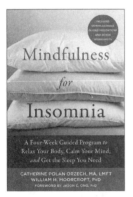
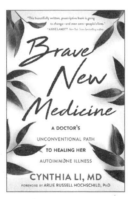
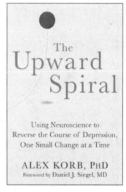

Register your **new harbinger** titles for additional benefits!

When you register your **new harbinger** title—purchased in any format, from any source—you get access to benefits like the following:

- Downloadable accessories like printable worksheets and extra content

- Instructional videos and audio files

- Information about updates, corrections, and new editions

Not every title has accessories, but we're adding new material all the time.

Access free accessories in 3 easy steps:

1. Sign in at NewHarbinger.com (or **register** to create an account).

2. Click on **register a book**. Search for your title and click the **register** button when it appears.

3. Click on the **book cover or title** to go to its details page. Click on **accessories** to view and access files.

That's all there is to it!

If you need help, visit:

NewHarbinger.com/accessories

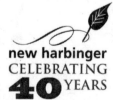

new harbinger
CELEBRATING
40 YEARS